A Lifetime in Medicine

by
Albert D. Roberts, MD

Copyright Page

G and J Publishing
Palm Springs, California, USA

Copyright © Albert D. Roberts, MD 2013

ISBN 978-0-9886295-5-4

All rights reserved. This book or parts
thereof may not be reproduced
in any form without written
permission from the Publisher

Visit Dr. Roberts web page at the
G and J Publishing Author's Gallery
www.GandJPublishing.com

In writing this book the author has tried to recreate events, locales and conversations from his memories of them and they are described according to his recognition and understanding of the events.

In order to maintain their anonymity in some instances he has changed the names of individuals and places. He may have changed some identifying characteristics and details such as physical properties, occupations and places of residence.

The views and opinions expressed in this book are those of the authors and do not necessarily reflect those of the publisher.

Cover design, editing and page layout by
G and J Publishing
www.GandJPublishing.com

Printed in the United States of America,
The United Kingdom and Australia

Acknowledgement

I retired September 30, 2004, intending to write an account of my then-54 years in medicine and including recollections from my physician-father's time going back to the '30s and '40s. Friends would say, "You've seen such changes, you should write a book!" I had long purposed to do just that, to recount my own education and career, beginning with the plywood shacks housing the nascent Southwestern Medical School of the '40s and '50s, to the immaculate towers of biomedical research, education and patient care that thousands and I now inhabit. Encouraged by my wife, I have written chapters on "Medicine Then and Now" and "Skeletons in Our Closet." I have also related the stories of a number of particularly memorable patients.

I made a good start back then, thinking the project might take a year or so. As it turned out, retirement lasted four enjoyable months, at the end of which I returned to work half time, and the writing became sporadic. Nevertheless, I had a first draft, mostly handwritten, some dictated, by 2008. Then calamity.

Because I can't really type and computers paralyze me, I required a stenographer who had big problems with my work output and, in effect, scrambled the manuscript. I rewrote much of it, making additions and changes as I struggled to work things out. Then a year or so ago, I and my project were rescued by my very capable niece, Helen Williams, a writer and editor with a tidy mind, good work habits and a tolerance for her uncle's idiosyncrasies. Also thanks to Helen's colleague at the Highland Park Independent School District, Elizabeth Perkins, for initially getting my book into book form.

I had initially worked with my high school and SMU classmate, Barbara Wedgewood. Barbara is a published author, teacher of creative writing and editor, successful at getting her best students published. She was able to purge some of my gratuitous literary flourishes, along with many semicolons and parentheses, attempting to mold me in the image of Strunk and White, and I am grateful to her for trying.

Most of all, I am indebted to my wife Diane, bearer of beauty, order and stability these 60 years, for encouraging my sporadic bursts of creativity and accepting my need for silence and solitude.

My most productive and enjoyable hours have been during our twice-a-year visits to Santa Fe. There, in the guesthouse of our dear friend Marion Turner, I have spent many hours in splendid isolation, my only companions the wind in the aspen, the songs of the birds and the scratch of my pen on paper. May the product of my labors justify her generosity.

    The names of my classmates, teachers, colleagues and friends are real. The names of the patients are not, except for Shanghai Jimmy and the Klemmes.

A Lifetime in Medicine

Chapter 1

Medical School

In the summer of 1950, I chose to attend Southwestern Medical School in Dallas in order to escape from my mother, who had moved to Houston with my youngest brother, John. I didn't base my decision to attend Southwestern on its reputation; in fact, it was a fledgling institution with a shaky identity. Rather, I knew that with both of my parents disintegrating, I had to make a better life for myself. So, despite the fact that the state's two more prominent medical schools – the University of Texas Medical Branch in Galveston and Baylor Medical School in Houston – had readily accepted me during my third year as an undergraduate student at Southern Methodist University, I decided on Southwestern.

My identity, my perception of myself as a distinct individual adult with goals, purpose, a projected career trajectory and perhaps the talents to achieve these things, began to gel on September 1, 1950, my first day of medical school.

With registration completed, about 96 men, boys, and four or five women assembled in the first-year classroom. The first item of business was the assignment of cadavers for dissection, one for each five students. Most of us already had formed ourselves into fivesomes, mainly based on undergraduate friendships and acquaintances, and we had scoped out what we hoped would be the best cadaver to dissect over the coming four or five months. So when our anatomy professor dismissed us that hot summer morning, there was a wild surge, Pamplona without the bulls, through the corridors to the anatomy lab, where we surrounded and claimed our preselected specimen. The idea was to get one in reasonably good shape, not too distorted by age, disease or trauma, such that body structures -- nerves, muscles, tendons, fascial planes and organs -- would not be too difficult to identify and dissect. Our cadaver was an old man slightly taller than average with distinctively aquiline features that were well preserved by the formaldehyde in which he had been immersed between death and dismemberment. We named him "the senator."

The anatomy professor was Dr. Bradley, a small, quick, diligent and friendly man who gave excellent lectures and dissection advice and instructions. Dr. Bradley died suddenly of a cerebral hemorrhage the following year. Local private practitioners and surgeons, who varied considerably in their degree of helpfulness, provided much of the supportive instruction in the dissecting room.

The other major courses that first year were histology, microscopic anatomy, biochemistry, neuroanatomy and physiology. Dr. Charles Gilderoy Duncan taught histology. He was at least 80, having come out of retirement to help this new medical school get under way. He was a silver-haired, avuncular man with amusing speech mannerisms. One of his sayings was, "You learn and forget, learn and forget again, and relearn, and then you die and forget everything." He was so endearing that the class bought him a hunting jacket and double barrel shotgun for Christmas. We didn't do that for any other teacher.

During that time, Southwestern Medical School was becoming part of the University of Texas system. A group of civic leaders, businessmen and physicians formed The Southwestern Medical Foundation in response to the Baylor Medical School's move to Houston in 1941 or 1942. Southwestern was still struggling in the early 1950s. But we students didn't know that. The school was in a World War II Army field hospital, a one-story, plywood structure identical to hundreds or thousands deployed in the war. A few years later, I served in one just like it in Fort Dix, N.J., while I was in the Army.

These hospitals were meant to last two or three years. By 1950, our medical school was notoriously decrepit, a continual maintenance challenge. There was no air conditioning except for a few administrative offices with window units, and insulation was minimal or absent.

There were no student desks. We sat in simple straight-backed chairs, our notebooks or clipboards on our laps.

December of 1950 was one of the coldest on record. For eight days before Christmas, the temperature did not get above freezing;

night temperatures were in the single digits. The steam heat system failed. Everything froze. The cadavers in the anatomy lab froze solid, and further dissection had to be abandoned. Members of the class of 1954 who chose orthopedics later had to arrange for a foot of their own to dissect because in January, we went straight to neuroanatomy. A couple of months later, another cold spell hit. On the day of our final exam, which included a "practical" — the identification of preserved tissue of all sorts — the specimens were frozen. We were all bundled up in such arctic gear as could be improvised, I in a bulky red and black Hudson Bay "Mackinaw" purloined from a relative who had gone to college in Wisconsin.

Students, Student Life

The class of 1954 was a strange mix. There were 100 of us, and the majority was veterans who had been to college on the GI Bill, ranging in age from mid-20s to late 30s. Most were married, some with children.

The class also varied greatly in educational background and scholarly ability. Since the school was still an upstart, it may have been the only one many of the students could get into. There were also some outstandingly gifted students who had chosen Southwestern. At least 10 became leaders in academic medicine and many more, leading practitioners.

But others were marginal, a few failed, and perhaps a dozen dropped out. Students from other states with only two-year medical schools filled some places — I remember South Dakota specifically — so we graduated at or near our original number. The graduation ceremony in June 1954 was held at SMU's McFarlin Auditorium. Outside there was a drenching downpour, well recalled because it briefly punctuated the terrible drought of 1950-1957, the years I was in training at Southwestern and Parkland.

Fraternity Life

We still had medical school fraternities in those days, even a vestigial fraternity rush. My first date with Diane Truett, my wife-to-be, was for a Phi Chi rush party at the old Dallas Country Club. I joined Phi Chi partly because it was my father's old fraternity. I followed his fraternity legacy and his medical legacy, as well. My father left his home in Stephenville, Texas, at age 20 to study at Baylor Medical College in Dallas in 1922. He always said it was to escape having to get up before dawn to milk the cow. He found out there were harder things than that ahead.

My roommate was Tom Murphy, a Navy vet slightly older than I was. We shared a spacious second-story front room in a handsome old frame house built in late teens or early '20s. It had a window that looked out onto Maple Avenue between Cedar Springs and McKinney. The house had two adjacent annexes and provided a home for about 35 unmarried men who shared and managed their own boardinghouse. Tom and I shared a bathroom with Jere Mitchell and Wilson Taylor our freshman year; subsequently, I shared a room in the annex with an upperclassman, Russell Turner, and Tom moved to an apartment.

Fraternity life was at times an amalgam of "Animal House" and "Doctor in the House." Purple passion parties were pretty wild, a shock to the unsuspecting. Guests were greeted in the dignified entry hall by a large washtub filled with grape juice and Everclear grain alcohol, bubbling ominously from the dry ice that had been thrown in. At the first such party Diane and I attended after I had pledged, Tom Murphy and I showed our new room to our dates. After we came back downstairs, a sophomore, Wade Greathouse, took me aside and quietly explained the rules: "No women in the bedrooms — if you want to fuck, there's a mattress in the attic." Also, if both doorways to the downstairs living room were closed, don't enter.

Wade, who died a few years ago, was a memorable character. An ex-Navy pilot from West Texas, he was part Indian and looked it. Standing 5'10", he looked like a prizefighter who had quit in time to preserve his rugged good looks. It seemed every time I saw him, four or five very young student nurses surrounded him. Once I watched while one tugged on the V of his scrub suit and stood on tiptoes to peer at his broad, hairy chest. This particular girl was the most beautiful of that year's crop, and he later married her.

Another character was Jack Elliott. Jack was tall, perhaps 6'2", dark and very handsome, resembling Lil' Abner. From a background that would now be called extremely dysfunctional, the closest thing he he'd had to parenting was the Marine Corps. He arrived at the Phi Chi house with a supply of olive drab Marine Corps underwear. He would place his grungy, stained socks and underwear in one of the bathtubs to soak with the other pieces there, removing the next set to wear after drying out overnight. All year long, Jack's underwear, socks and sundries filled that tub. He believed in gratifying his basic urges before studying. Typically, this meant a visit to Frankie's Rendezvous Lounge at the corner of Maple and McKinney, followed by a quick turn with one of the many young women living in old apartment buildings across the street. I remember watching him cross the street to the frat house and pause by the front bushes to lower his fly and eject a just-used condom. Then he went upstairs to cram a few hours.

The Phi Chi boarding house had a mascot, an ancient rust-colored terrier mix named Terry. Terry's exact age was unknown, but tribal lore placed him in his mid-teens when I was a freshman, and he lived several more years. Terry was quiet, patient and tolerant. At one of the raucous purple passion parties, I watched one of the seniors, belly full of firewater, crash through the front screen doors, lurch across the porch, collapse over the porch rail, fall through the bushes and lie motionless. Terry sat by him all night until he awoke.

Phi Chi had weekly chapter meetings, usually desultory and poorly attended affairs, but from time to time we had guests, ranging from the relatively exalted (Dr. Milfred Rouse, President of the AMA) to naked dancing girls. A great favorite was Dr. Vincent Vermooten, a sixtyish South African urologist. Bald, slight, slope-shouldered, and mildly cross-eyed, he resembled the writer S.J. Perelman. He showed us two 8-mm movies from his homeland. One showed two lions engaged in glorious, combative foreplay. It was so violent, it seemed one or both of the creatures would perish. The end, the climax, in sharp contrast lasted only a few seconds: a shuddering orgasmic spasm, then quick collapse into blissful supine post-coital torpor.

Dr. Vermooten's other film documented a mass circumcision of Zulus. Outdoors, somewhere in the veldt, stood a long line of robust, young black men, stark naked. Each in turn was placed on a sturdy wooden table and held fast by four strong men in white coats while two doctors performed the ancient rite. One would hold the penis erect by clamping the end of the foreskin with surgical forceps while the other snipped it off. No anesthetic; it lasted only a few seconds. Released, the victim would then walk knock-kneed away clutching the bandaged member. Today it seems barbaric -- racist, even -- to watch or admit to having watched such a spectacle. The doctors in the 1930s believed they were performing an important public health service, and contemporary studies confirm that circumcision decreases the frequency of cancer of the penis and the transmission of venereal disease, including HIV.

But still, it says something about the times that no one in our crowd thought to ask whether the Zulus submitted voluntarily or were somehow coerced, or perhaps even paid.

Another favorite was Dr. Tate Miller. Dr. Miller, an internist and gastroenterologist then in his 70s, was a large, bald, gregarious man with a barrel chest and raspy voice, the result of decades of heavy smoking. A popular raconteur, Dr. Miller was invited to the frat house for his humorous tales as well as his wisdom about medical practice. After supper ended, Dr. Miller would push back from the table, fire up a cigarette, inhale deeply and address the 30 or so medical students thusly:

"Young gentleman, people often ask me the secret of success in medicine, and I tell them, 'the practice of medicine is not unlike the sport of duck hunting, and the rules are three: First, step boldly to the fore. Second, shoot every time anybody else shoots. And third, take credit for everything that falls.' "

Just a few steps away from the Phi Chi house, at the corner of Maple and McKinney, stood the Rendezvous Lounge, always called Frankie's after the small, olive-skinned, mustachioed proprietor. Frankie looked Sicilian and liked to imply that he had been in the rackets. He certainly looked the part. The lounge was a small, low, white frame house. Inside, there was a bar with seven or eight stools and a few booths and tables where Frankie served beer and wine. It was still illegal to sell liquor in public establishments, although you could bring your own bottle. The little lounge was a regular hangout for medical students and a few neighborhood characters. One such was known as Mrs. Benton (not her real name). She was well past any possible bloom of youth she might have once had and was none too fastidious in appearance. For some desperate students, she was the bedmate of last resort, alleged to acquire a phantom allure after 6 or 8 beers. I recall one morning after we'd all partied following a big exam. A classmate woke up his three roommates, sobbing remorsefully.

"What happened, Elroy?"

"I can't (sob) talk about it."

"Better tell us."

More sobs. "I screwed Mrs. Benton. We had a few beers. She started to look better and we went to her room. Then, she took her corset off. Oh, it was awful, but by then I couldn't stop. God, I feel terrible."

The boarders at the Phi Chi house ate well, and the house was reasonably well kept. The cook was named Maurice; there was also a housekeeper. Both were black and homosexual, although not overtly, at least not while on duty. Maurice was intelligent, fastidious and perceptive. The housekeeper, Maurice's consort, didn't say much, but did his work. His predecessor had been a large black woman named Agnes, who had a syphilitic aortic aneurysm, a common condition in those days. One day it ruptured, and she died instantly.

We made up our own beds, if they were made up at all, and looked after our own laundry and personal things. During the week, the house was mostly quiet after supper. Everyone studied. Friday and Saturday nights were for partying, except before exams.

The big freshman-year courses besides anatomy, histology, and neuroanatomy were biochemistry and physiology. All courses included didactic lectures and laboratory practicums. The physiology course was particularly basic to the foundations of medicine and very well taught by Dr. Robert Lackey. Dr. Lackey gave lucid and well-organized lectures. He was strict and firm, stringent and fair in his grading -- no such thing as grade inflation back then. A "B" was honors, and an "A" was rare. Dr. Lackey leavened his lectures with dry humor. I recall him referring, straight-faced, to the "magazine reflex" as a reliable stimulus for defecation. For those of us who later entered one of the nonsurgical specialties, physiology was the most important course of the first two years. I was content with my B.

The summer of 1951

In that dim past, there was no school from June 1 to September 1. I spent that summer in Houston with my mother and youngest brother, John, at her jewel of a little house on Inwood Road in River Oaks.

I was in love with Diane and wanted to be near her, but I had no money and no job in Dallas. So we agreed to be "unpinned" for the summer, and I spent the three months in Houston working as a lifeguard at the Shamrock Hotel.

The strain of this summer-long separation, while leavened by Diane's visits and letters, interrupted a relationship that had been constant and intense ever since we clicked on that first date. This slim, auburn-haired girl with the big brown eyes and terrific shape was different from anyone I had dated before. She was smart, had a wide range of interests, and was as stimulating to talk to as she was to look at. Although we both attended Highland Park High School, we did not meet until the spring of my third and last year at SMU, when she returned from her freshman year at Mary Baldwin. I remember the first time I noticed her. She was horseback riding with one of her high school boyfriends. I said to my brother, Bob, "That girl knows how to sit on a horse."

Isolated in my lifeguard's tower in my shades, whistle, hat, and green trunks, I had quite a varied scene to observe at the Shamrock. The notorious wildcatter Glenn McCarthy, the inspiration for Jett Rink in Edna Ferber's "Giant," had just built the hotel. The 50-meter swimming pool was the first Olympic-sized commercial pool in the U.S. and was part of the Cork Club, which offered private membership, but was also open to hotel guests. The deep end was 25 feet. There was a 10-meter diving platform and one-meter and three-meter diving boards. Young divers abounded, both novices and advanced competitors. Serious divers frequently used the pool to practice for national and international events.

Across the pool from my observation perch stood the Cork Club cabanas for members, guests, and trysts, a dozen prime call girls in view. I recall a day when McCarthy was hosting a very young Nicky Hilton. This was before his marriage to Elizabeth Taylor. Midday, McCarthy lined up the girls in their tiny bathing suits for Nicky to inspect. There was a longish picnic table, spotless white linen, laden with a choice of beverages, though bourbon was the favorite potion in those days. McCarthy, big, broad shouldered, and noticeably fender-bellied, filled a quart pitcher first with ice, then with Jack Daniels Black Label, which he finished – alone. I don't recall what Nicky drank or which girl he chose.

The lifeguard job was the ideal therapy for recovering from the exhausting freshman year and preparing for the next.

Home life was far from ideal because of Mother's binge drinking and squandering of her divorce settlement. This was the last time I was ever to live in the same house with my mother. She had moved to Houston following her divorce from her second husband,

John R. Moroney, who was a brilliant, flamboyant lawyer and a severe manic-depressive. He committed suicide a few years after the divorce.

My mother was a famous beauty who retained a good part of her looks until the end of her life. Sensitive and intelligent, she was the standout in a rambunctious family of eight children, seven of whom survived childhood. She was the only one to attend college, a year at SMU. Her drunken, dissolute, sometimes violent father contracted to build the sidewalks on the university's quadrangle, and mother's tuition was part of the payment.

The move to Houston was a desperate attempt to rebuild her life, and it marked the beginning of a long downward spiral.

So the summer passed. After work, I would drink a beer or two, play the guitar, talk with 12-year-old Johnny, or visit Aunt Merle and Uncle Dale. I read a lot, as I always have done.

I didn't save anyone from drowning that summer. I don't remember even having to pull anyone out. The only challenges came when drunken conventioneers (doctors were the worst) would shatter glass at the poolside or try to climb the 10-meter tower. No, the only person I saved was myself.

Sophomores

I returned to Dallas and to reality that September rested, tanned and fit. Diane put my ATO fraternity pin back on, and we have been together as often as possible ever since. The sophomore year I remember as mainly drudgery, relieved by friendships and by Diane and her parents. The Truetts frequently had me over for dinner – the best food I got in those years – but I still felt that Diane's mother, Mayme, did not really approve of me.

The big second-year course was pathology. Both the course and the academic year were dominated by two very different and antagonistic personalities, Atticus James (Jim) Gill and Ernest Eric Muirhead. Dr. Gill had been afflicted with tuberculosis of the spine — Pott's disease — and gallantly bore its deformity, short stature and crooked spine. He was a handsome, fine-featured man who spoke in a melodious voice and wore a three-piece suit year round, the vest covering his back brace. His lectures were masterful. The hour devoted to Pott's disease remains hallowed in the memory of all who heard it.

Equally admired but for different qualities and on the whole by different factions of students and faculty, was Ernest Muirhead. Later, when he was at Baptist Memorial Hospital in Memphis, he was called Eric.

Dr. Muirhead was tall and strong, with clear blue eyes and graying russet brown hair. In contrast to Dr. Gill's precise adherence to the known facts of classical pathology, Dr. Muirhead was a visionary driven by almost compulsive speculation and imagination. His lectures could be enthralling. His delivery involved dramatic physical gesturing. "Big spleen!" he would exclaim, illustrating its size with his large hands, and then "Big liver!" his hands holding the imaginary organ on the other side. He was also passionate about research and pursued the elusive, putative renal antihypertensive factor to the end of his career.

The rivalry was always apparent and lent drama to the otherwise rather dreary second year. The inevitable clashes worsened after Dr. Gill became dean of the school and Dr. Muirhead the chairman of pathology. Eventually, Dr. Gill removed Dr. Muirhead from the chairmanship. Two or three years later, to the dismay of his many friends and supporters, Dr. Muirhead departed. He remains in the minds of all who came under his spell almost a legendary figure, not least because we continued under his tutelage on the hospital wards where he was one of the first clinical hematologists. He made teaching rounds at the bedside, where he was a thoughtful physician, as well as an inspiring teacher.

Friendships begun the freshman year solidified the second and were instrumental in our survival of the physical and psychological stress of long hours in uncomfortable lecture rooms and constant study. My closest friends were Floyd Rector, Andy Gwynne and Dick Portwood. Floyd, from Lubbock, Texas, was a brilliant student. His wife Margie was a commercial artist who supported them and later their girls, through medical school. Both have had remarkable careers, Floyd as a medical scientist and Margie as an artist. Dick Portwood, a Navy vet from San Antonio, and his wife, Ginny, were also close friends. Andy Gwynne, whom I had known at SMU, deserves a chapter devoted to him alone. Andy was, to put it gently, disorganized. His intellect was mercurial and wide-ranging; an amazing disarray of facts in all fields: science, history, literature. This information he could access at random, especially after a few drinks, when his conversation could be fascinating, but seldom in a sustained, orderly way. Thus, his academic standing, while he was never in any in danger of failing, never reflected his native intelligence.

Everyone has a friend like Andy. They appear from time to time in literature, like Charles Stringham in Anthony Powell's A Dance to the Music of Time. They sparkle, dazzle and flame out, but remain precious in memory, and we are richer for having had them as friends. Andy was given to bursts of generosity; a treasured possession of mine is a 1911 Britannica given me by him many years ago. Not a part of this nucleus but equally close was David Haseltine, honored in memory. We had been close since high school; he was a year ahead in the Highland Park High School Class of 1946. At SMU, I pledged to ATO because of David. We were then classmates in medical school because he finished four full years at SMU, having decided to attend medical school to train as a medical illustrator. He had a strong artistic bent, but soon was on the main pathway to becoming a physician.

It is hard to convey the effect David had on those of us who knew and loved him, men and women alike. He was an extraordinary blend of strength and sensitivity. His most notable physical feature was a tremendous physique. He was a terrific swimmer and natural athlete but forbidden to compete in sports because of a heart murmur. A highly malignant brain tumor tragically shortened his life. He had his first seizure during our third year. In retrospect, I think there was some deterioration in his cognitive skills after that, but he endured to marry, father a daughter and complete part of his internship at Grady Hospital in Atlanta.

His deterioration was very hard to bear. I was in the hospital room with him a few hours before he died. He is mourned by all who knew him well for the warmth of his friendship and the strength, breadth, and depth of his character. A number of us have sons named David.

Toward the end of our second year, I think we all felt battered by the incessant didacticism, constant study, memorization, and the physical and mental constriction imposed by the arduous curriculum. We survived, thanks to our friendships. I remember spring of 1952 when David, Andy and I took sandwiches to nearby Reverchon Park, cutting class for the afternoon, strolling or lying in the grass in the gently warm spring sun.

The Introduction to Clinical Medicine provided a blessed respite from the lecture halls. We put on our first white coats and learned to use stethoscopes, ophthalmoscopes, otoscopes, reflex hammers and tuning forks. We went to the bedside in small groups, where the art of physical examination came to life.

My instructor of physical diagnosis was Roger Unger, who was in private practice at that time. He later became a world-famous researcher in diabetes and lipid metabolism. Roger was directing a U.S. Public Health project to study the accuracy of the glucose tolerance test in diagnosing diabetes in the general population. As I recall, he found a 40% "crossover" rate on repeated testing: 40% of initial positives became negative and vice versa. Roger was, and remains, totally unaffected, open and accessible. He taught us easily and well. He was my first close encounter with a sort of well-educated, highly intelligent Easterner who would become a major factor in the school's subsequent success. At that time, he was not on the faculty, but was a volunteer teacher, along with many of our teachers, especially during the clinical years. I admired this group and their academic and social sophistication, which soon inspired me to buy my first Ivy League tweed jacket, plain front grey flannel trousers, Irish poplin ties, and blue or white button-down Oxford shirts.

There was another memorable encounter, equally influential in a somewhat different way. Bill Reynolds was a practicing internist, specializing in gastroenterology. He was partially paralyzed by bulbar and spinal poliomyelitis. Though he got around quite well with only a cane, he was frail. His impairment did not detectably slow him. He was thoughtful and patient, a fine teacher. There is an additional reason why Bill is so clearly remembered: I mean the site of the tutorials.

In the early 1950s, the old original Woodlawn Hospital was a one-story, white frame building situated on a slight hill on Harry Hines Boulevard where the Children's Detention Center now stands. It was the charity hospital for indigent tuberculars. The location was intended to be salubrious, with its location upland from the Trinity River, catching southern breezes in what was still a fairly rural area, though only a mile or so from downtown Dallas. During this era, antibiotics were still fairly new, and tuberculosis was treated with prolonged bed rest and lots of fresh air. As I recall, there were a couple of wards and perhaps a few small rooms for sicker patients, but the sickest patients, the ones most likely to die, are the ones I recall most vividly. They lay in cribs, pale, apathetic, hollow-eyed, and near skeletal. Cribs were cubicles placed on the periphery of the building, isolated from an inner hallway by a wall with a port for passing in food and medicine and removing wastes, used bedclothes, and dirty dressings.

The upper half of the outer wall of each cubicle was a large, hinged wooden shutter, like they used to have at summer camps, to be raised and lowered by rope and pulley. So it was there at the old Woodlawn that we first donned gowns, masks, and gloves, and Bill Reynolds patiently taught us to examine chests, review the chest radiographs (X-rays) of ravaged lungs and learn therapeutic treatments, which have since been abandoned. One procedure involved inserting a tube between the lung and the chest wall (pneumothorax) or into the peritoneal cavity (pneumoperitoneum) and pumping in air. This would decrease the lung volume relative to the blood supply in the hope that this would close the tubercular cavities and speed healing.

At Woodlawn and at Old Parkland (now called Woodlawn) we, in our new white coats, were mistakenly called doctor for the first time. Those of us who had not seen combat were confronted for the first time with the sick, the dying, and death. Bill Reynolds continued to practice another 30 or 40 years despite his frailty, imperceptibly weaker as time went by, until a late phase when he went down fairly fast. Perhaps this was late progression of the postpolio syndrome.

Remembering Bill Reynolds evokes a stream of thoughts and memories, including those of young doctors in training who fought their own illnesses. Until the 1950s, tuberculosis and poliomyelitis were probably the most common serious afflictions. However, various other kinds of physical and mental collapse were common: depression, alcohol and drug problems, and a rare suicide. One or two developed tuberculosis during the course of training, at least prior to 1950. I recall the previously mentioned classmate Andy Gwynne, who was diagnosed with tuberculosis during his residency in pathology. Also, the wife of one classmate contracted polio but recovered completely.

In the class ahead of us, the class of 1953, Gene Waterman had had bulbar polio and was left with some problems swallowing at times, but he was fully functional, an excellent student and house officer.

Less fortunate was Larry Vivrette, in an earlier class, probably class of '51. One summer day, likely after a day and night on duty, he and fellow students were drinking beer at the old Vickery Park swimming pool, near where Presbyterian Hospital now stands. Suddenly, Larry could not swallow. When he tried, the beer came out through his nose. He was admitted straightway to the polio ward and was dead by morning.

There were many doctors in the decades and generations before me who had had bouts with tuberculosis, also known as the white plague. We were all exposed to it repeatedly through inadvertent contact with undiagnosed cases (and doubtless through lapses in isolation technique), and the circumstances favored susceptibility. We were frequently exhausted, often sleepless; our nutrition was not all great, either. Most of us smoked cigarettes. The classical phthisiologists (from the Greek phthisis, wasting) were almost all recovered tuberculars; among them were older friends and mentors like John Chapman, Frank Carman and Elliott Mendenhall. Not all who had the illness became chest specialists, of course, for example, Billy Oliver, long one of Dallas' leading internists. Billy believed that his bout with tuberculosis was divine intervention because it was through that illness that he met his lovely wife, Chris, who was one of his nurses. Some of these doctors had been in the sanitarium for up to six years. As they were allowed to become gradually more active, they helped with the care of other patients. Many of them went on to become phthisiologists, chest specialists, and forerunners of today's pulmonologists.

The writer Walker Percy was diagnosed with tuberculosis during his pathology residency at Bellevue in New York City and spent two years in the Trudeau sanitarium at Saranac Lake in upstate New York. There he read philosophy, epistemology and Kierkegaard, and thus became Walker Percy the writer. I don't suppose I am the only one who has sometimes wondered what it would be like to have a mild case of something for long enough to enable the pursuit of alternative interests or passions, then to recover, or perhaps be reborn like a butterfly from its chrysalis, into a new existence.

The end of the second year, for some of us the least enjoyable, finally came. Despite sound teaching and some vivid personalities, my friends and I felt thoroughly depleted, relieved to see the end of the term, and grateful for another summer's rehabilitation. There were the welcome moments of levity, one supplied by the wife of Andres Goth, the professor of pharmacology, wise, kind and thoughtful toward the students. Andres and his wife were Hungarian and both spoke with an accent, hers stronger than his was. Dr. Goth told the story that one day he and his wife were discussing buying a new car. He said he would

A LIFETIME IN MEDICINE

like a Volvo. She said, "Andres! Do you know what that means in Hungarian?"

Those first two summers of the medical school years were of vital importance to me because those three months of relatively salubrious existence facilitated my recovery, not merely from the normal exhaustion of medical school terms, but also from my imagined fatal illnesses. Cliché as it is to joke about the medical student who fears he has every disease he studies, it is not so funny when you have as onerous a bout with imaginary illness as I did.

In the spring of my freshman year, 1951, I became aware of increasing fatigue and lassitude. I had experienced spells like this going back many years, but now I was a medical student, and very much focused on disease. At first, I was sure I had malignant melanoma. Several of my numerous moles (junctional nevi) were removed during my freshman and sophomore years, and pathological examination found them to be benign. Every time I noticed a new mole, I'd think, "Well, this is it."

Once, I found a batch of flat, black spots on my left forearm and dashed over to see Dr. Dan Gill, a splendid surgeon and cousin of Dean Jim Gill. Dr. Gill was skeptical that these spots were anything, but to humor me, or perhaps to get rid of me, he removed one or two for pathological examination. Negative. Nothing there. In a few days, the remaining spots went away completely. As it turns out, I had splashed a few tiny drops of silver nitrate on my arm during a laboratory experiment, and they went unnoticed until they turned black.

So the melanoma hypothesis became untenable. I did not lose weight, my liver did not fill up with metastases, and my studies went reasonably well throughout all of this.

But the lassitude and fatigue persisted, greatly aggravated by the "fever study," which went like this: One of our teachers wanted data on diurnal fluctuations in body temperature. My fellow students and I were enlisted to take our own temperatures four times a day -- rectally. I had not yet learned, and we were not informed, of the normal three or four degree variation from early a.m. 'til evening, say 96 degrees lying in bed before breakfast; 99.4 in late afternoon; after a cigarette and a cup of coffee, easily 99.6 or 99.8, technically "fever." Severe anxiety can make it worse. So I became obsessed with this, taking my temperature hourly sometimes, surreptitiously (not rectally, of course) in class, growing more and more anxious as the afternoon temperatures climbed, fearful that something was terribly wrong. I began to poke myself. By then, we were taking pathology, and this sharpened my focus. To my deepening concern, I found fairly impressive lymph nodes under my jaws, in my armpits, a few small "shotty" ones above the collarbone. Naively, I asked a third year medical student to confirm my "lymphadenopathy," which he did, then said carelessly, "You have Hodgkin's disease," which in those days proved fatal in months to a few years.

So now I knew my fate: I was to die of Hodgkin's disease. Easter Sunday, 1952, Highland Park Methodist Church, Reverend Marshall Steel preaching, remains especially vivid in memory: I thought it would be my last Easter. I could even imagine Jesus up there in the stained glass, behind the choir, beckoning.

I did not speak of this to Diane, friends, or family. Instead, I became a regular attendant in the student health service, presided over by patient and kind Dr. John Vanatta. We ran tests. It did not help that I tended to run a somewhat higher lymphocyte count in the peripheral blood, or that one day in the student hematology lab my own blood sample showed 98% lymphocytes -- a fluke or staining error, as it quickly developed. Nor was I reassured when our Chief, Dr. Muirhead, consoled me with, "Why don't you worry about stomach cancer? You could have that too, you know."

Dr. Muirhead's version of shock therapy was opposite to the response I got around about 10 o'clock one night, when I desperately called up Dr. Jim Gill at home. He was patient and reassuring, and he calmed my panic, telling me that he understood, that he had "been there."

The sophomore year was the worst, but again, summer brought salvation. The sun, exercise and rest worked their cure. The illness never returned in that guise except for brief flashbacks, again usually associated with late winter or early spring and fatigue. Once in my third year, Dr. Vanatta sent me to someone in our then rather weak Psychiatric Department.

The consultation did not go well. The psychiatrist, obese, epicene, slothful, lolled behind his desk, smoking cigarettes while regarding me passively through half-closed eyes, saying nothing. Although I was by then disposed to accept a psychological basis for at least some of my symptoms, the encounter so revolted me that the reaction effected a substantial "cure."

A LIFETIME IN MEDICINE

The definitive diagnostic test, of course, would have been a lymph node biopsy. This was never done. And almost 60 years later, the nodes are still there, unchanged.

Despite these distractions, with more help from Diane and her family and kind teachers and robust friendships than I have ever acknowledged, I survived the freshman and sophomore years, even made all B's – solidly placing me in the upper third of my class. There is little doubt in my mind that this experience deepened my understanding and tolerance and made me a better physician. A further benefit has been that, having faced imaginary death off and on for a couple of years, I have never really feared it again.

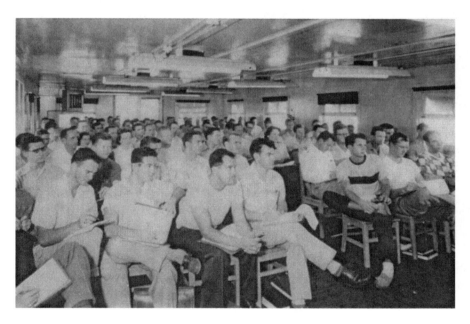

The freshman classroom, 1950. I am third from the right in the first row.

ALBERT D. ROBERTS, MD

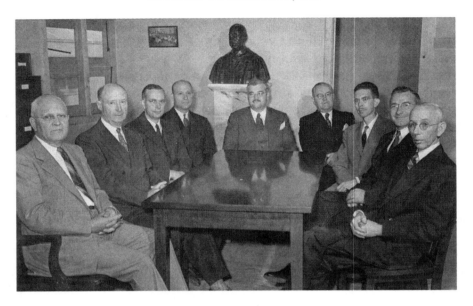

The original full-time faculty, 1943. From left, Charles G. "Daddy" Duncan, histology, embryology; George T. Caldwell, pathology; Joseph Hill, clinical pathology; Robert W. Lackey, physiology; Donald Slaughter, dean; Lewis Waters, medical illustration; Herbert C. Tidwell, biochemistry; MacDonald Fulton, bacteriology, and William W. Looney, gross anatomy. All other positions were filled by part-time town men. Dr. Looney, right, instructed my father at Baylor Medical School in Dallas in the 1920s. After the first quiz, he advised my father to return to his father's drugstore soda fountain. At the end of the year, my father finished first in anatomy.

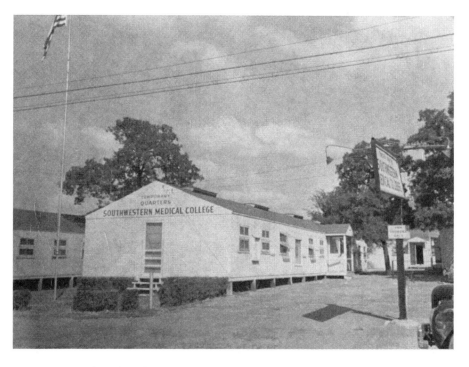

"Temporary" housing for the new Southwestern Medical School, 1943-1957. We nicknamed them the shacks.

Chapter 2

My Annus Mirabilis

The third year was my Annus Mirabilis; the summer of 1952 was its prologue. My job as lifeguard and swimming instructor at the old Dallas County Club, a bunk at the ATO house at SMU, and a beautiful girlfriend -- what a healing antidote to the gruesome life of a medical student! I took breakfast every morning at the counter of Skillern's Drug Store in Highland Park Village across Preston Road from the DCC. Invariably, breakfast was the 19-cent special: one cup of coffee, one egg (usually fried), a piece of toast and one piece of bacon. I took lunch in the basement of the DCC with the other employees and could choose from the daily menu or a sandwich or burger. Most days, I had either two cheeseburgers or two triple-deck ham and egg sandwiches on whole wheat. When they fired the head lifeguard, I was promoted and spent the last six weeks of summer working 8 a.m. to 10 p.m. I took supper at the club as well.

In just a few months, I went from employee to member. If you married a member's daughter – which I was soon to do – you could join for $400 (Diane's parents must have loaned us the money). I had a special relationship with former fellow employees. For many years thereafter, a waiter would sometimes, when serving the drinks at our table, say to me, sotto voce, "Leave a little in your glass, Doc."

I was paid $75 a month, but expenses were negligible, and with added income from swimming lessons, I was able to save enough money for a down payment on a nice engagement ring for Diane. I had a nice 1950 four-door Plymouth, tan, 85 horsepower. I had also escaped my mother, whose deterioration continued. Nothing spoiled the summer.

A LIFETIME IN MEDICINE

Among the children I taught are a few who remain sharply etched in my memory. Foremost was an undersized boy of 11 or 12, badly crippled by tuberculosis of the spine (like Dr. Jim Gill, but worse). Not only was his back deformed, damage to the spinal cord had also weakened his legs. He had curly blond hair, blue eyes, and smiled nearly all the time, scampering about like a little spider. He loved the water and learning to swim more than any child I ever knew. His parents were not at all well off. Friends who were club members provided lessons and guest privileges. After that summer, I did not see him again.

I also taught the two roly-poly sons of Dr. Pierre Girard, the Chairman of Orthopedics at Southwestern Medical School. The boys, about 4 and 6, did not readily take to the water. But, at the end of two or three weeks, they could swim the length of the pool -- necessary for successful "graduation" -- and were reasonably safe and confident in the water.

I taught several 2- and 3-year-olds. Around age 2, there is a window when children are easily brought into the water and taught. About 2½ to 3, fear comes into play, and learning becomes more difficult until age 5 or 6.

I developed my own teaching methods, having myself never been formally trained. Some of my more challenging pupils were rejects from a well-established swimming teacher of the time, "Pop" Kitchens. It is only a slight parody of Pop Kitchens' method to say, as one of his former clients told me, "He will throw your child into the water and if he makes it to the edge by himself, Pop will say 'I can teach your son to swim'." Otherwise, not.

So I became a self-taught remedial swimming teacher. In late July or August, I gave thought to making a little more money by working at Parkland Hospital. The only job for which I was remotely qualified was night ward secretary on the polio wards. Polio was widespread again that summer, and the wards and rooms were full. I recall two large wards, each with about 10 iron lungs enclosing bulbar polio patients. There were also a few smaller rooms with one to four patients in various stages of decline or recovery.

My job required me to collect vital signs at each patient's bedside and record them in the charts. As this entailed close contact, I wanted to wear a protective outer garment, as did the nurses and doctors, though that was not a requirement for ward secretaries. Failing to locate an isolation gown or a scrub suit, I finally donned a green garment that seemed adequate. This action provoked odd looks, and at first, furtive comments from my coworkers. Soon the night administrator arrived. He was a young man named Rod Bell, who later became president and CEO of the Presbyterian Hospital System. Rod was about 6'5", not yet fat. Looming over me, he said my costume was "inappropriate" and then ordered me to remove it. I rather piously refused, stating that I, too, needed protection, adding that in a few hours I would be teaching swimming lessons to children. An annoyed and frustrated Rod Bell turned on his heels and grumbled away.

Shortly thereafter, my friend, Wade Greathouse, by then an experienced senior student, happened along, took one look at me, and said, "You look ridiculous. You're wearing a nurse's dress. Take that thing off!" So I did, chastened and humiliated. After a few nights, I gave up. Working two jobs was not worth the fatigue and the time away from Diane.

The autumn of 1952 was the springtime of my life. I had endured the dreary and didactic preclinical years. It was not all bad, of course. Some students, those comfortable with the rote memorization and passive regurgitation of received wisdom, thrived. Others of us survived to emerge out of the cramped classrooms and on to the hospital wards where we saw real patients, real world issues, and prompt and visible consequences of our actions. Above all, for me, it was a heady atmosphere of fresh challenges that came every day, opportunities to collect, synthesize and apply information, and to observe outcomes. There was close contact, one-on-one or in small tutorial groups, with a variety of mentors ranging from Interns and Residents to vigorous professors in mid-career and wise, distinguished senior physicians.

I was fortunate in my first assignment: The Internal Medicine Service at the old McKinney, Texas, Veterans Administration Hospital, 45 miles north of Dallas. Like the medical school, the McKinney VAH was housed in a World War II Army hospital building -- one story, plywood with large wards, long hallways. Students and some Interns and Residents were housed in the Bachelor Officers Quarters (BOQ) next to the hospital, 75 or 100 feet across a parched lawn from the main buildings. Each of us had a small room like a monk's cell: a narrow bed, small table, straight-back chair, lamp and desk. The bathroom and showers were down the hall. In those days, there was nothing to do in

A LIFETIME IN MEDICINE

McKinney or if there was, I didn't know about it. We took our meals in the mess hall; the food was pretty good by those days' standards. There was nothing much to do but study. I cannot imagine a more favorable hatchery for a future clinician.

I should explain here that the McKinney VAH and the one south of Dallas at Lisbon, Texas, were Dean's Hospitals, a category developed after the war to provide quality care for veterans. Chiefs of service and staff physicians were medical school faculty appointed by and serving at the pleasure of the medical school dean. The McKinney Internal Medicine Service was presided over by the revered Dr. Ben Friedman. Wise and meticulous, Dr. Friedman exemplified the best qualities of his generation. The mid-20th century now seems in retrospect the late flowering of the Oslerian model, which was embodied in the person and career of Sir William Osler (1849-1919), the most influential physician of his era. This was the tradition of the bedside teacher, when "Grand Rounds" really were bedside visits led by the chief throughout the hospital. Laboratory resources were meager. What mattered most were the careful, nuanced medical history and the meticulous physical examination. This required using all the senses and plenty of time and led to a diagnosis, prognosis and treatment program. Dr. Friedman was such a doctor, as was his friend and mentor, Dr. Tinsley Harrison.

Dr. Harrison left Southwestern before I arrived as a freshman, but he returned to lecture several times while I was there, a great showman on rounds, inspiring to students and young physicians. He edited Harrison's Principles of Internal Medicine, still perhaps the preeminent textbook of Internal Medicine. The 13th and 16th editions sit by my left elbow as I write.

Other "giants" of that era were Paul Beeson, Paul Dudley White, George W. Thorne, Dana Atchley, Robert F. Loeb and Sam Levine. A good many of these famous doctors passed through Dallas as visiting professors. I recall Wesley Spink from Minnesota speaking on brucellosis and hearing him urge students to develop for themselves one or two such lifelong fascinations. William Dock, I remember, speculated that his Jewish patients were deliberately overeating and under exercising because they (unconsciously?) wished to die so their children could inherit. George W. Thorne from Harvard lectured for an hour on what he considered the best single laboratory test -- the lowly sedimentation rate. I was not impressed. William Bean, the white-haired, courtly longtime chief at Iowa, talked for an hour about his thumbnail. These men represented the old order, white males who were swiftly to be displaced by a new order, doctors more rooted in scientific investigation and objective data, much less on intuition, personality and cogitation. More empiricism, less authoritarianism. Among these visiting professors were two strong exceptions to the white male predominance of that era: thyroidologist Rosalind Pitt-Rivers and liver expert Sheila Sherlock, both British.

Dr. Tillett came in the '50s to describe his life's work on treating empyemas, infected fluid between the chest wall and the lung surface, with the enzyme streptokinase. Dr. Tillett was near the end of his career. He endeared himself to me by initially rambling on a bit, a few minutes of irrelevant chatter, necessary he said, after all these years and hundreds of talks, to calm himself down, to let the nerves subside. I read in the March 3, 2005, issue of the New England Journal of Medicine, an article on the same subject, streptokinase in empyema; not effective. Tillett not cited. But Tillett's cases, at the dawn of the antibiotic era, might well have benefited.

Tinsley Harrison's tenure at Southwestern was not a serene one. He could be charismatic. He attracted a coterie of bright young men wherever he went, many still alive and loyal to his memory. He sponsored several of them into the new National Institutes of Health; others, with his influence and support, obtained residencies and fellowships at prestigious northeastern programs, such as Massachusetts General and Peter Bent Brigham, despite having matriculated from an obscure little medical school. But Harrison was self-absorbed, irascible at times. As time went by, he drank more. He engendered controversy among the small faculty and hostility from the leaders of the "town men," the unpaid volunteer teachers whose continued support was vital to the school's survival.

Frustrated, Dr. Harrison left Southwestern to become the chairman at Birmingham. On his last night in Dallas, a half dozen of the city's leading internists hosted a farewell dinner for him. The honoree had drunk a good deal of bourbon by the time he proclaimed that Southwestern would never be a first-class medical school because the Dallas doctors were all sons of bitches. "Well, Dr. Harrison," replied one of the hosts, "when you get on that train for Birmingham tomorrow, there will be one less son of a bitch."

A LIFETIME IN MEDICINE

In their own ways, Dr. Harrison and Dr. Friedman were outstanding examples of the previously mentioned noble Oslerian tradition. Dr. Osler was the dominant clinician of his era. He defined the internist-educator: thoughtful, cultured, keenly observant, and focused on meticulous examination, diagnosis and prognosis. Osler himself was something of a therapeutic nihilist, which was all to the good. Prior to the first decades of the last century, most of the popular nostrums were ineffectual or harmful.

Dr. Donald Wayne Seldin, who irrupted into the Dallas scene in 1951, embodied the dawn of a new paradigm. He was still anchored to the bedside, clinical care and teaching, but much more rooted in laboratory investigation, using powerful new methods of chemical analysis to explore more deeply the biochemical and pathophysiological basis of disease. Medicine was about to become much more science-based, and Dr. Seldin, perhaps more than any other individual in the last century, would make it so.

Thus, it was that I was present at the denouement of the old and the conception of the new, like one of those cherubs in a Baroque allegorical painting. I first encountered Dr. Seldin at his regular weekly teaching conference at the McKinney VAH where I was a raw third-year student, a "clinical clerk" in the parlance of the day. This was the fall of 1952. We were assembled, sitting there in straight back, wicker-bottom chairs. Presently in came Dr. Seldin, just 32, six feet tall, slender, well dressed and dazzling.

As Interns presented case histories, Dr. Seldin fidgeted. He would ask a few critical questions, and then the patient would be brought in for a brief examination. After the patient departed, Dr. Seldin would start the discussion. His voice was rather high-pitched, with a strong New York accent, strange sounding to flatland Texas boys like me. His sentences were rich and finely wrought, rolling along into comely paragraphs and precise syntax and grammar. His style was not so much formal or pedantic as passionate, persuasive and bristling with facts. He paced all the while. If there was a blackboard present, data soon covered it.

That's how it would go. He was threatening, exhilarating, challenging, exciting, and full of information. We had never seen anyone remotely like him, nor experienced such impact. For the first time, I was confident that I had made the right decision in going to medical school, and I never again wanted to be anything but an internist. Dr. Friedman, quiet, gentle, probing and equally scholarly, afforded a balancing contrast to Dr. Seldin. He was particularly good at extracting the telling detail in a patient's history. One day one of the medical Residents was presenting the case of a man with tertiary syphilis who had repeatedly denied ever having the primary lesion, the painless ulcer or chancre that the World War I veterans called a haircut. After a few of Dr. Friedman's casual, indirect questions, the patient abruptly said, "You know, Doc, I had syphilis when I was in France."

We saw many cases of tertiary syphilis in veterans, aortic insufficiency and neurosyphilis, seldom to be encountered again in private practice. I remember with affection the big open wards, even some individual patients. My first assigned patient was a black World War I veteran, accustomed to medical students and tolerant of us. My first morning on the wards, I was told to draw my patient's blood for lab tests. The fact suddenly struck me that I had never learned how to draw blood. Luckily for me, my patient had forearm veins like hoses. I must have shown some trepidation because he asked me something like, "Do you need a little help there, Doc?" And -- this is what I was like in those days -- I replied, "Do you think this is the first time I have ever done this?" and hit the vein with my first shot.

There was another World War I veteran named Earl Hart. Although he wasn't my patient, I remember him well. He had wide-open aortic insufficiency, head bobbing with every heartbeat (de Musset's sign). But that was not the reason he was there. His problem was chronic intractable diarrhea, as resistant to diagnosis as it was to treatment. Earl was an engaging man, and one day while we were visiting, I asked if I could examine him, and he obliged. I found hard, pea-sized lymph nodes in odd places such as along the border of the pectoralis muscles. That evening, as I was browsing through journals in the small hospital library, I discovered a Journal of the American Medical Association (JAMA) article on small cell lymphoma involving the small intestine, and it described patients with features like Earl's. The next day at rounds, I pointed out the nodes to Dr. Friedman, who gave me credit for close observation. Those eight weeks in the fall of 1952 were my baptism into clinical medicine. I was, in fact, totally immersed and emerged reborn.

We had another eight weeks of medicine wards, this time at Parkland, which was considerably more demanding than the VAH. Between the departure of Dr. Harrison and the arrival of Dr. Seldin, the

A LIFETIME IN MEDICINE

school had slumped and was, in fact, on probation for a while. There were a few months when the full-time faculty in Internal Medicine consisted exclusively of Dr. Don Seldin. Soon others came, Louis Tobian, Alvin Shapiro, and Leonard Madison. Also making teaching rounds were Ernest Muirhead (Department of Pathology) and Arthur Grollman, Chief and sole incumbent of the Department of Experimental Pharmacology. Volunteer faculty did much of the ward teaching. Many of the leading practicing internists made teaching rounds -- gratis -- and contributed greatly. They were truly indispensable.

During my years at Parkland, I had as town attendings, J. Morris Horn, Billy B. Oliver, Mike Scurry, Baldy Brereton, Sam Shelburn, Jack Edwards (who taught me electrocardiography), Jim Herndon, and Howard Heyer. Among other excellent volunteer teachers I did not encounter on my rotations were Al Harris and Paul Thomas. All of these men practiced general internal medicine, although a few designated themselves as subspecialists: Dr. Heyer, Cardiology and Dr. Brereton, Gastroenterology.

The house staff was small and uneven. After Dr. Harrison decamped, quality declined. Dr. Carl Moyer, chairman of Experimental Surgery, had left, as had Gilbert Forbes in Pediatrics, as well as the dean, George Aagard. These men had given the new school real distinction, and their departure threatened its survival. After several tergiversations, Dr. Seldin finally made a lifetime commitment, resolving himself to stay, recruit and build the program.

There were a few good medical Residents along with a couple of duds left over from the pre-Seldin hiatus. The chief resident my junior year was Ben Bridges (Tyler, Texas). There were also David Miesch (Sherman, Texas) and Richard Hunter (Dallas). These three were among the most skillful physicians I have known; all became distinguished practitioners.

This was the year and the environment that made it all come together for me. I cast aside personal fears and cares, threw myself body and soul into it, learned rapidly, read everything and finished with an "A" in Medicine. I did reasonably well in the other courses, Surgery, Obstetrics and Gynecology, Pediatrics, and Psychiatry, and finished third in my class that year – the highest I got.

Another vivid personality was Dr. Gladys Fashena, professor of Pediatrics, quondam Acting Chairperson. She was a strong presence --

handsome features, clear diction, and a commanding personality. She was firm and exacting but empathetic; no trace of meanness, something that could not be said of some others. At her famous and feared conferences with students, new cases were presented and students selected at random for close and sequential questioning. When my turn came, I got everything right except the actual diagnosis -- the baby had presented with neonatal vomiting, and the cause was congenital adrenal insufficiency. Dr. Fashena said it was "a good junior-level performance."

Dr. William Mengert, a rigid martinet who modeled himself on the 19th-century Prussian tradition, commanded OB-GYN. Widely recognized in his field, he was the founding chairman of his department in the upstart school and important in establishing its reputation. I remember him as often harsh and cruel in word and deed, capable of tormenting subordinates. My experience was, overall, pleasant, owing to fortunate friendships -- Douglas Haynes, the vice chairman (and the only other full-time OBG faculty that I recall) and some fine Residents, including Jim Goodson and Tom Nabors.

Tom and his wife Connie took a special interest in us and had us to dinner. For a short while, Diane worked as his receptionist, and she decoratively painted the restroom at his office.

Doug Haynes developed alopecia areata. We all thought Dr. Mengert had him tearing his hair out, figuratively as well as literally. One night during my senior year, he invited Diane and me to his apartment for an evening. I had neglected to tell Diane that half of Doug's hair was missing. As he turned his head to wave us in, she reacted with open-mouthed astonishment, which was brief and, thankfully, unobserved. Then he sat us down, handed us each a large glass of bourbon and ice, and treated us to a memorable evening of grand opera, technical musicology, and even a bit of early karaoke.

Diane and I were married December 22, 1952, after a courtship of two years, eight months. It was at the start of our Christmas vacations, hers from teaching third grade at Longfellow Public School. We had a beautiful wedding a Perkins Chapel on the SMU campus and an elegant reception at the Dallas Country Club. It was the last such reception at the old brown frame two-story clubhouse where I had worked as lifeguard and swimming instructor the previous summer. We spent the first night in our new furnished apartment on Douglas Avenue (one year's rent was a wedding present from Diane's parents). The next morning, with $300 in my pocket, we got in the 1950 Plymouth and drove to Shreveport, where we spent the night on the way to our honeymoon in New Orleans. Diane and her family provided a nurturing balance that I had never experienced before, setting the foundation for my "annus mirabilis."

In the spring of the junior year, I began to plan how to spend the summer. We would need income because Diane had become pregnant in February, so she would not be teaching in the fall. There was no summer school. I thought it would be wonderful to work in Dr. Seldin's laboratory. My friends Andy Gwynne and Floyd Rector told me I was foolish to even think Dr. Seldin would have any use for us. But I worked up the courage to ask him, and in fact, Dr. Seldin was eager to have us do a summer of research in his laboratory. Miraculously, he even had a little money: $200 a month for each of us. Considering our apartment was $90 a month, that was considerable money. We were not lab technicians -- we were research fellows! Floyd, Andy, and I worked directly with Dr. Seldin. Other classmates doing research projects that summer were Norman Kaplan, future hypertension expert, and Bob Cade of Gatorade fame and fortune.

Floyd and I worked together on the effects of potassium deficiency and carbonic anhydrase inhibition on ammonia formation, acidity and electrolyte composition of blood, urine, kidney and muscle. It was a rather ambitious project, entailing a lot of work. We performed all aspects of the experiment, all the chemical analyses. I tube fed the rats. Twice a day I donned thick gloves, removed each large, angry Sprague-Dawley rat from its cage, restrained it, and then inserted a wooden dowel with a hole in it between its jaws. The feeding tube went through the hole and, with luck, into the stomach. Skill, persistence and patience were required, and I was bitten once or twice a week. Every day, we collected and analyzed the rat urine and sterilized the equipment. At the end of 14 days, I exsanguinated the rats and analyzed their blood samples. This process took all day and well into the night.

Floyd's task was even harder. He stripped muscle from the carcasses, reduced the samples to ash in an oven, and then ran a chemical analysis on each specimen. All of this could take upwards of 30 hours. We cleaned up after ourselves, as well.

We had one of the early Weichselbaum flame photometers, a forbiddingly huge apparatus that had to be fired up and standardized each time we used it. Spending long summer nights in a small, un-air conditioned room, my reward was not only the accurate data, but also the beautiful colors of sodium and potassium flaming in the night.

An old man who wore his battered hat askew and drove an old mule-drawn wooden wagon began appearing on the days our experiments ended. He would pick up the rat remains from the trashcans outside the small shack where we kept the rodents. Apparently, he fed the scraps to his hogs. Floyd Rector tells the story that one day, as he was dumping the residue, the hog farmer rolled up, surveyed the scene, and remarked to Floyd, "You boys may be real smart, but you sure don't seem to know much about taking care of rats."

Floyd and I were in daily and almost nightly contact with Dr. Seldin, whose energy and enthusiasm propelled us along. He seemed to require no sleep. One of the best features of that summer was the long conversations over coffee at Lucas' B&B Cafe on Oak Lawn, sometimes at 1 or 2 a.m. Dr. Seldin would check on us late at night in the lab and drive us to the café in his feeble little Prefect (an English Ford that was briefly imported during the '50s). That summer of 1953 was the middle of the great seven-year drought that hit Texas from 1950-57. We didn't much mind or even notice the heat; neither our homes nor work places were air-conditioned. We were fully acclimated. Toward the latter part of the summer, I had a recurrence of my lassitude and apathy. I no longer attributed it to physical illness, though it would be many years before I recognized it for what it was -- depression. My work performance declined, perhaps not dramatically so. I always muddled through those bouts with no spark and little joy. The other complication was summer school. This onerous circumstance came about because the Texas Legislature, in its great wisdom, had ordained that every graduate from a state school -- graduate schools included -- must have taken and passed an undergraduate course in Texas history. Southwestern had become a state school after I completed my premed requirements, so although I was a senior medical-school student, I had to complete the two-semester undergraduate course.

I returned to SMU during the summer of 1953 to take the first semester, which was taught by Dr. Ballard, whose American history course I had greatly enjoyed just four or five years before. This time around, after three hard years in medical school, I was shocked that Dr. Ballard had become a tired old prof, just getting through the hour. I found the students to be intolerably jejune. I survived the first semester, collected my C, took the second semester by correspondence, and squeaked out another C. This ill-conceived requirement was rescinded almost immediately after I complied.

Firstborn

Diane went into labor in November 1953. We met Dr. W. K. Strother at Baylor Hospital, and I sat with Diane as labor progressed, about six hours. I had expected to go into the delivery room with Diane, but Dr. Strother surprised me by saying it would be better if I did not. Then came a long night of waiting, dozing alone in a dark room and smoking many cigarettes, apprehension dimly working its way up through a fog of fatigue. Finally Dr. Strother appeared, his habitually jovial demeanor now deeply somber: Diane was fine, and the delivery was completed without complications, but Brenda, our baby girl, had severe congenital defects, hydrocephalus and spina bifida. Dallas' leading neurosurgeon of those days, Dr. Albert D'Errico, was summoned next day. Dr. D'Errico arrived in the room, told the nurse to turn the baby over, glanced briefly at Brenda and pronounced her inoperable. Then he said she would not live a year. Our pediatrician, the eminent and much-admired Dr. Robert Moore, agreed. We found him distant and unsupportive, and he offered no guidance. When our two other children, son Truett and daughter Hillary, came later, we went to Dr. Floyd Norman, another leading Dallas pediatrician and the husband of the great Dr. Gladys Fashena, whom I have already mentioned.

It was an awful time for us, a crisis. I was a third-year medical student with no family support. Diane was an unemployed schoolteacher. We made the decision not to bring her home. Diane and I left the hospital and drove Brenda to "Angels Unaware," a home for such infants, which was located on Maple Avenue near Oak Lawn. I provided medical services in return for free medical care, and "made rounds" regularly, advising on common illnesses and problems—though the staff undoubtedly knew as much as I did. Most of the patients were grossly deformed with tiny bodies and huge heads that housed brains that could not develop. But there was no suffering that I could see, and they were all lovingly attended.

Dr. Strother had suspected Brenda's deformity by the third trimester, when it was clear that she was breech, her head up under the right rib cage and rapidly enlarging. But he said nothing to us. Things were done that paternalistic way in those days. Extracting the baby without damage to mother or baby was a considerable technical feat. Brenda's head grew rapidly for the first few months. Then it stopped growing. She survived her first year with no illnesses, then her second, and her third. Although Brenda lived to her mid-50s, her mental age never progressed past six months. All those years, she required constant care, first in privately owned sanitaria, then in state schools. The last several decades, she was at the Denton State School, situated on a beautiful, quiet campus and staffed by devoted caregivers. I visited her every few months. The decision we made in November 1953 enabled us to have a normal life, two wonderful children, and now two beautiful granddaughters, Truett's daughter, Sara, and Hillary's daughter, Carina.

Diane's parents helped us get through the rest of medical school, enough to live on until Diane could return to work, which she did as secretary in the Parkland ("the Old Parkland") Blood Bank, directed by Dr. Ruth Guy, who became a good friend. Diane registered donors and did clerical work. One of her duties was to go to the opposite end of the hospital to the emergency room to retrieve unused blood. This entailed exposure to a fair amount of gore and some really bad sights, sounds and smells. I was assigned to the E.R. much of the time and would fetch the blood for her. Despite the hardships, Diane loved being a part of student and intern life. She earned her "Old Parkland" creds, and has her share of colorful tales to tell.

Seniors

The final year went by very quickly and was enjoyable, except for a dismal experience in Pediatrics, where Residents, who I thought were mostly a bunch of dim bulbs, did most of the teaching. After my successful third year and my summer research project with Dr. Seldin, I thought I was pretty hot stuff. I was a bit arrogant, sometimes obnoxious. The pediatric Residents didn't like me, and I didn't like them. I was lucky to get a C in the course, which probably knocked me out of the top 10 in my class. The joke about the Class of 1954, the "illustrious Class of 1954," as Dr. Carleton Chapman called us, was that out of a class of 100, there were at least 20 in the top 10. The

A LIFETIME IN MEDICINE

Pediatrics imbroglio also removed me from contention for the Ho Din Award, the annual recognition for the outstanding member of the graduating class. Years later, I was told that my name had been put forward, but Pediatrics vetoed it. The award went to my close friend, David Haseltine, who deserved it.

There is this one story worth recounting from my otherwise miserable fourth-year tour on Pediatrics. I was working in the charity clinic at the old Children's Hospital at Maple and Wellborn. A woman came in with her nearly 3-year-old son. They made an amazing contrast. She looked like a subject from Richard Avedon's catalogue of trashed-out rednecks, a little taller than 5 feet, lank blondish hair, pale blue eyes, and the skin and mucous membranes of chronic anemia. She looked hollow-eyed and exhausted, very thin and stooped, with some teeth missing. She was not yet 30. Her son was an infant Hercules, muscular and vigorous with bright blue eyes, perfect white teeth and a halo of blond curls.

About the time I asked what the trouble was, Hercules thrust his strong little arm into his mother's loose shirt, extracted a withered breast, and began to suck robustly.

"I waited too long to wean him," came the resigned explanation.

This is not something I heard from someone else or read in a novel by John Steinbeck or Erskine Caldwell. I could do little. I tried to help with whatever had prompted the visit, and they left. I rotated off service and never saw them again. She had said they were too poor for bottled formula.

After Pediatrics, the rest of the senior year went well. On Obstetrics, I delivered about 50 babies, often unassisted except for an obstetric nurse. And there were also exciting times in Surgery. Several episodes stand out in my memory.

Dr. William Mengert, the Bismarck of OB-GYN, decreed that there would be postpartum follow-up house calls by an OB-GYN resident, a nurse and a fourth-year medical student. The policy would permit earlier release from hospital and allay possible hospital-acquired complications. This allowed us to see how our patients and their families actually lived -- in shacks and hovels, mainly in West Dallas. We got a firsthand look at deep poverty and deprivation; this was a half century ago. We would enter a darkened room to find a teenage mother lying on a sofa, cot or pallet on the floor with some relatives and the baby nearby. Fathers were rarely seen. We'd check the vital signs -- any fever? Check the lochia -- normal secretions or purulence? Baby nursing? I remember treating a frightened teenage Hispanic mother who was living in a shack/half-cave dug into Trinity River clay. There was no water, electricity or bathroom facility of any kind.

This program ceased with Dr. Mengert's departure. Too bad. I hope it was as beneficial for the patients as it was for me -- I've never forgotten what it felt like to be there, and the memories form my social and political orientation to this day.

In Surgery, we had excellent faculty and Residents. Ben Wilson was chief, Jerry Stirman and Morris ("Fogey") Fogelman good teachers. My surgical team had Bob Stewart (long dead from malignant hypertension) as third-year resident and Ernie Poulos, second year. How we worked! It was the time of "see one, do one, teach one." This hoary maxim was literally true and could have been coined at the Old Parkland. I clearly recall an all-nighter when I found myself all alone in an operating room, dawn's first light creeping through the east windows, closing the belly of a knifing victim whose abdomen Bob, Ernie and I had just explored. They had moved on to the next case, taking the nurse and anesthetist with them. I was left to finish up, with luck, before the anesthesia wore off. On another night in the spring of 1954, young Bob Potter (not his real name) and his pals got into a bar fight. Bob got a bullet through his neck, severing a large artery at the base of his skull. He was brought to the E.R., exsanguinating, bled out, deep shock, pulse and blood pressure unobtainable. Somehow, we got a line in a vein, pumping saline until the blood arrived, then transfusing as fast as we could, barely keeping up with the pumping artery. A severed artery retracts, and this wound was deep. In the operating room, Bob Stewart dissected and probed, probed and dissected. We were running out of blood. We decided to tie off the vertebral artery on the side of the bleeding, gambling that the other vertebral would supply enough blood through connections at the base of the brain to prevent a massive stroke. The vertebral was ligated, but still the hidden artery pumped. We were out of blood -- 26 pints gone. Fishing around for the gushing artery was like trying to grab an eel in a muddy hole. We had been on duty over 20 hours without rest. Bob Stewart's shoulders slumped with exhaustion. Ernie Poulos, who had been first assistant all this time while I held retractors and wielded the suction, said, "Let me have a try." He took a hemostat, thrust it into the wound, and clamped. The bleeding stopped, and vital signs stabilized. Bob Potter made a complete recovery. Months later, when I was an intern with an M.D. after my name, I saw him skipping across the parking lot, leaving the clinic.

"Hey, Bob!"

"Hi, Doc!"

Then there was Art Livingstone. Dr. Livingstone, white-haired and around 50, had been a GP in Alberta many years before coming to Parkland for a residency in Urology. He was slow and deliberate in speech and movement; our nickname for him was "Living Stone." One day Dr. Livingstone was checking my skills at the prostate exam. An elderly black man was bent over the exam tablet, rear end exposed, awaiting his exam. Dr. Livingstone handed me a glove. It was a size small.

I said, "Dr. Livingstone, I will need a larger glove. You must remember you're in Texas now."

Art's measured reply: "Well, yes. The assholes are bigger in Texas."

Many years later, I told that story at a medical meeting in Banff, where I was a speaker. I was told that Dr. Livingstone was alive and well, enjoying his retirement. My last rotation of the senior year was on Thoracic Surgery. The chief resident (seventh year) was Ben Mitchell. The other resident was Pil Woon Hong, from South Korea. A splendid surgeon and ferocious Ping-Pong player, he returned to Korea to become one of the foremost surgeons of his native country. Our "town attendings" were Dallas' foremost thoracic surgeons of that time, Drs. Shaw and Paulson. Bob Shaw was highly revered and had trained with the legendary Evarts Grahame in St. Louis. Paulson was mercurial.

I was the only student, and my duties seemed to have no end: complete admission histories and physicals on all patients; draw blood for tests; start IV's; pass catheters; assist at surgery (suction and retractors again; some suturing) and, finally, make ward rounds with the team. We were on duty every day and every other night. I might have been averaging four hours' sleep a day, but I felt little or no fatigue. It was the last week or so of medical school, things were going very well, and I had that exhilaration that lies beyond fatigue. In short, I was in an exuberant state.

Then one day I was dashing along the halls at Parkland, chatting with a classmate when he said, "Your eyes look yellow. Do you feel all right?" A glance in the mirror confirmed a yellowish tint.

Fear and exhaustion came in waves. Was it metastatic melanoma? The dreaded Hodgkin's disease? What if it was merely hepatitis, which would require a few weeks of bed rest? Suddenly, hepatitis sounded oddly appealing. Next, I made the physician's classic mistake; I ran a test on myself. I went to the laboratory and did a bromsulphalein test, a long-obsolete measure of liver function. The upper limit of normal was 5%. Mine was 30%! I ran to see Dr. Leonard Madison, a brilliant young internist who had joined our faculty. Dr. Madison examined me, highly skeptical of my presumed illness. Out of caution, he admitted me to the hospital overnight for testing. I told Diane about it, reassuring her that although it could be something serious, fortunately, we had caught it early.

I spent the night in the hospital's single air-conditioned patient room, which was reserved for metabolic studies. Luckily for me, there were none in progress. At dawn my classmate, Floyd Rector, came in and drew many tubes of blood. And then I waited. I had to admit I felt pretty good after a sound sleep in an air-conditioned room, but as the day wore on, my anxieties grew rapidly. Finally, a little after 5 p.m., in came Dr. Alvin Shapiro, another recent addition to the faculty, who told me to get up, get dressed, and go home. "Your tests are all normal," he said. "The BSP is not 30%. It's 3%. I'm signing you out "acute subluxation of the decimal point."

I made a miraculous recovery. The yellow tint was little fat pads adjacent to the iris.

Graduation

The ceremony was held at McFarlin Auditorium on the SMU campus. I recall that it rained heavily – a rare event during the seven-year drought – and that the Ho Din award went to my friend, David Haseltine. Diane's parents were proud of me and of having helped Diane and me get to this point in our lives. Almost nothing else do I recall, certainly not the name of the speaker. We did stand for the President of the Dallas County Medical Society to administer the Hippocratic Oath, the 20th-century version, which, unlike the classical version, did not require us to "swear by Apollo," or forbear to" cut for the stone."

A LIFETIME IN MEDICINE

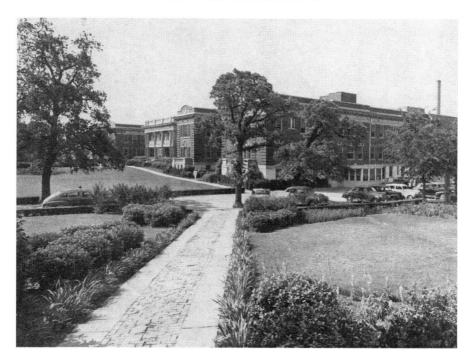

Hallowed ground, "Old Parkland," 1911-1954, as viewed from the student nurses' quarters in the 1940s.

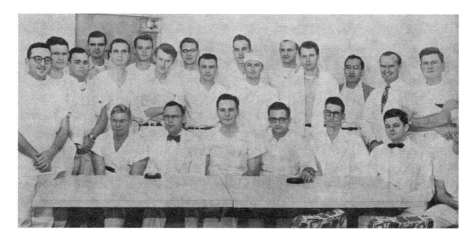

Interns, 1954-1955. From the student nurses' annual. I am fourth from the right, second row.

Chapter 3

Internship and Residency: Tales of the Two Parklands

Bliss was it in that gray dawn to be alive,
But to be young was very heaven!

Wordsworth's lines are apt. Like the French Revolution, medicine was exhilarating, terrifying at times, and bloody. An acquaintance of those days told me that I "burned with a bright blue flame," which is what G.B. Shaw said of his sister at her cremation. It was also a fair description of my zeal and determination. On the night of July 1, 1954, on the first day of my internship, my flame nearly went out. I lost a patient and thought it my fault.

The patient was a boy of 15 with severe thrombocytopenic purpura, practically no platelets; bruises from failed blood clotting covered his body. During the day, he developed an intracranial hemorrhage and lapsed into coma. Nothing was helping. The last order I wrote before going home was for intravenous 5% glucose in water, but I unintentionally wrote it in an ambiguous way, and the nurses interpreted it as distilled water. Distilled water given rapidly intravenously in sufficiently large quantities causes hemolysis – the rupture of red blood cells – a serious and potentially fatal reaction. The boy died during the infusion. The resident on duty called me at home to inform me, his tone somber and faintly accusatory.

The first person I called was my father, who was a plastic surgeon in Fort Worth at that time. Doctors of my father's generation had a saying: "Just wait 'til you've killed your first patient – that's when you find out whether you're a real doctor or not."

A LIFETIME IN MEDICINE

That is what my father said to me then. It was said in an understanding and sympathetic way, a tough-minded man's way of being supportive.

Although the statement sounds outrageous to contemporary ears, it embodies a truth. Things do go terribly wrong sometimes, and one must accept and live with guilt and a sense of failure and yet learn and persevere.

Cold comfort it was to me then. I thought I had killed a boy and was not at all sure that I was a doctor, after all. I then called Dr. Leonard Madison, who was my ward attending physician. He and Dr. Seldin were both at a party. Both spoke to me at some length, first getting the particulars (how much distilled water, and at what rate?), then forcefully reassuring me that I had not killed the patient, who had died of his disease and not of the medication error.

There would be other times in the future when things would go badly and I would blame myself and feel wretched, but I have never felt as shaken as I did that first night on duty as an M.D.

I spent the next three years as intern and resident, initially at the "Old Parkland," at Maple and Oak Lawn. Then in October of 1954, we made the momentous move to the new Parkland Memorial Hospital, a couple of miles away on Harry Hines Boulevard.

The old hospital still stands today. For a long time, it was desolate and derelict, but sturdily resistant to decay. Now, it has been beautifully renovated and put to new purpose by the Trammell Crow Group. Still, a moment's reverie (or better yet a quiet stroll around the old campus) evokes a tumult of vivid memories of crowded halls, large open wards, the chaotic Emergency Room, along with their sights, smells and sounds.

Built in 1911, the Old Parkland replaced the white frame 1890s building that had been the first Dallas County charity hospital. It had no direct relationship with a medical school, as far as I know, before becoming the primary teaching hospital of the new Southwestern Medical School, formed when Baylor Medical was enticed away to Houston in the early '40s.

Many of Dallas' leading physicians were private practitioners who contributed care. Their payment came with the prestige and unparalleled experience that such positions provided. These included the Chief of Surgery Dr. Lee Hudson and Dr. John Vivian Goode. Dr.

ALBERT D. ROBERTS, MD

Goode was a legendary martinet who was trained by Halstead at Johns Hopkins Medical School in Baltimore.

Once when he was doing an abdominal operation, some troublesome complication arose, perhaps a torn artery or penetrated intestine. Surgical assistants, nurses and a throng of observers surrounded the operating table. Suddenly, Dr. Goode commanded, "Somebody grab that retractor." A bare hand and ungowned arm stole into the sterile operating field. Dr. Goode, rigid and pale, stared fixedly straight ahead and said, "Get him out of here. I don't want to know who he is, just tell him to get out of my operating room."

Later, when Dr. Goode was not appointed chief, he left the faculty.

My father interned at Parkland in the 1920s when the salary was zero and some Interns supported themselves by selling their monthly whiskey prescription allotments ("spiritus frumenti") to pharmacists for $100, according to my father. This was illegal, of course, but unlike many activities related to Prohibition, it provided a positive benefit to otherwise destitute Interns.

With the formation of the Southwestern Medical School affiliation, the department chiefs were all full-time salaried faculty members: Internal Medicine, Surgery, Obstetrics/Gynecology, Pediatrics, and Psychiatry. Patient care was supervised, and medical students and House officers were taught by both full-time faculty and unpaid volunteer private practitioners. It was 1954, and our chief was the young Dr. Donald Seldin. Six of the eight straight medicine Interns that year were the same Parkland medicine Interns whom Dr. Seldin inspired as third-year and fourth-year students. We considered ourselves something of an elite cadre. The eight were Charles R. Baxter, Jere Mitchell, Dick Portwood, Andrew Gwynne, Floyd Rector, Tom Hair from South Carolina, John Rumsfeld from up north somewhere, and me. All but Tom and John were Texans who were educated in public schools.

I have heard Dr. Seldin say that when he left Yale for Texas, people told him he would never find good students, but what he found was a group that would equal the best anywhere. Baxter, Mitchell and Rector went on to brilliant careers in research and academic medicine, and all achieved substantial success. My own contribution has been more devoted than distinguished. Baxter, Hair, Gwynne and Portwood are all dead. There were also outstanding future physicians among the rotating Interns. The late Bob Cade became famous for inventing Gatorade while working at the University of Florida Medical School in Gainesville. Another future luminary was Norman Kaplan, now a world leader in hypertension. Donovan Campbell became a pioneer in anesthesia for open-heart surgery. Robert K. Bass was a leading Dallas internist until his retirement; and the late John Gunn went on to become an outstanding orthopedic surgeon and early leader in total joint replacement.

In the years before The Millis Report (1966), formal training on Internal Medicine was four years -- a year of rotating or straight medicine internship, then three years of residency. Subsequent to 1966, it took three years to become a general internist, with many or most continuing on for another two to four years of subspecialty training.

Our first-year duties were divided into inpatient wards, outpatient clinics and the Emergency Department. The following years added rotations through the subspecialty consultation services: Cardiology, Infectious Disease, Pulmonology, Endocrinology, and Nephrology. Neurology was then a division of Internal Medicine. Until the late '50s, we lacked full-time faculty in Rheumatology, Allergy-Immunology and Gastroenterology; private practice consultants filled those roles. Much of the teaching was still provided by "town men" (not a woman among them), who made rounds on the inpatient services for a half-day, twice a week. They heard case presentations, usually went to the bedside and discussed the diagnosis, work-up and management. They had little or no responsibility for actual patient care, and they varied widely in capability. Some were superb teachers and role models; others were simply something to be endured.

The full-time faculty members were nominally responsible for patient care, but the Residents really managed things and did a substantial part of the teaching. Supervision was typically casual and indirect compared to today's stringent requirements. The attendings taught us the theory and practice of Physik – clinical medicine and its biomedical scientific basis – at the bedside and in small-group sessions organized around the day's case presentations, while all direct patient care and responsibility devolved to the house staff. This configuration was a major attraction to the more aggressive and ambitious medical student, and remains so today, though greatly altered by the many layers of rules and regulations that now constrain medicine at all levels.

ALBERT D. ROBERTS, MD

I believe the personal care that patients received then may have been better overall than it is today. The great scientific and technical innovations, such as total joint replacement, open-heart surgery, effective medication for many common diseases, have been to some extent offset by changes in the economics and social structure of medicine. Physician authority and responsibility have been redistributed. Economic pressures determine career choices and affect medical decisions more than they once did. Physicians are beset by regulations of Mandarin complexity.

In our training, standards were taken to be the highest attainable, consequent upon our own zeal and determination to do the best we could in every situation, but due also to fear -- fear of the consequences at failing to perform well. Charts were scrupulously reviewed on the thrice-weekly faculty ward rounds. Most dreaded -- and most educational -- was the Friday noon Death Conference. There, mistakes of any kind, instances of simple carelessness or sloppy thinking, were mercilessly exposed and ventilated, and perpetrators were excoriated. These meetings were known as "Indigestion Rounds."

This categorical insistence on a meticulously thorough and complete work-up on every patient set a high standard of care and a rigorous educational experience. The same atmosphere prevails in most determinedly academic environments today, but it is not an altogether admirable practice. In their zeal to dress the chart and avoid criticism, many House officers overdo it, ordering too many tests and diagnostic procedures, and not applying enough critical thinking. Sometimes the patient can get lost in the extravagantly expensive process. Fear of litigation is tangential. Mainly it is the Zeitgeist – tradition, habit and mindset – at all levels. The parsimony of our forebears had its merits.

In 1954, they paid us $25 a month; later in the year, it was raised to $50. Hospital meals were free, and the food was execrable. Once or twice a week, the main course in the hospital cafeteria was bean burgers: limas or some other leftover mashed into patties, fried and slapped between stale buns. The food improved somewhat in the new hospital. But our favorite spot was the short-order cafe in the basement, which stayed open until midnight. Intended for visitors, it was, through some administrative oversight, free for house staff, along with our regular cafeteria meals. It was a splendid thing for the team to descend at 10 or 11 p.m. for a cheeseburger or two and a milkshake.

When the administrators figured out what it was costing, they shut down the cafe.

There was also a separate dining room for house staff and faculty, which we used for mealtime meetings. It was open all morning, and the ladies auxiliary volunteers supplied doughnuts and coffee. There we would all mingle informally after morning rounds, the only place where Interns and Residents from all the specialties could socialize. When I was Chief Resident, I could do a day's work of organizing and supervising in an hour or two – and in pleasant surroundings. The administration closed that down, too, claiming it was unfair to the nurses and other employees.

Until the 1950s, it was customary for hospitals to provide living quarters, the traditional compensation being food, housing in the hospital, uniforms, laundry and pocket change. In the Old Parkland, the quarters were on the top floor of the East wing, converted in-patient rooms with double-decker beds and a telephone. Toilets and showers were down the hall. There were only a few female Residents, and they were offered rooms in the nursing students' quarters.

Most of us were married and had apartments, thanks to working wives, but a few still lived in the hospital. It is hard to believe now, but for a few weeks, one of the surgical Residents at Old Parkland lived with his wife and two children in an inoperative elevator, cadging meals from the cafeteria kitchen.

Throughout the summer of 1954, we were on duty every other night, meaning that we were off maybe 12-14 hours out of 48. Usually you could get a few hours' rest, though not always. We performed many tasks now done by paid staff: starting IV's, placing nasogastric tubes and urinary catheters, drawing blood for lab tests and doing some lab tests ourselves. We had a small lab on the sixth floor where we could do blood counts, urinalysis, bacterial stains, and spinal fluid exams. Most doctors have lost these skills now, putting them at the mercy of lab techs. Much was lost when the immediacy afforded by these labs was removed, owing to liability issues and quality concerns on the part of the Pathology Department.

The seven-year drought burned on. Old Parkland lacked any air conditioning except for the administrative offices and blood bank, and the same was true of the New Parkland for several years. We admitted many heat-stroke victims, patients brought in unconscious and sweatless with body temperatures 106-110 degrees and even higher.

ALBERT D. ROBERTS, MD

We immersed them in tubs of ice. Most died; some survived, only to have second heat strokes while in the hospital. One night in the mid-1950s, I admitted five heat stroke cases. All eventually died of their complications.

One summer we were in a grisly competition with St. Louis for the most heat stroke deaths. St Louis won by a slight margin topping out at over 100 cases, probably due to greater humidity.

By the end of August 1954, some or all of us were near the breaking point. I certainly was. I went to Dr. Seldin, who was aware of the situation. After that, we were on every third night, and it was never quite so bad. Still, the E.R. assignment continued to be every other night for several years throughout my residency, which ended when I was drafted in July of 1957.

Heat stroke was not the only signature illness of the early to mid-1950s: the other was poliomyelitis, which abruptly disappeared with the advent of the Salk vaccine. The mass inoculation effort enlisted all the House officers. In 1954, I went with a group of Interns and nurses to Hillcrest High School, where we injected thousands of people. The sight of so many persons, types never before encountered in other venues, who appeared not to have been out of the house or even seen daylight for years, struck me: pasty white, corpulent, clumsily coping with the unfamiliar scene.

Then quite suddenly, gone were the daily and nightly polio admissions, the urgent tracheotomies, and iron lungs, polio wards staffed by teams from the Polio Foundation, and the deaths or partial recoveries.

There was one episode, far from typical, that veterans of those days will tell when we gather. On a hot night in August of 1954, a man was brought to the E.R., no history provided, apparently paralyzed, speechless and barely breathing – clearly bulbar polio. A tracheotomy was swiftly done, and he was transported to a polio ward and placed in an iron lung.

The pulmonary team arrived the next morning. The patient was slid out of the respirator for a brief examination, whereupon he was found to be not in the least bit paralyzed. The doctors speculated he might be a catatonic schizophrenic. At that point, the subject placed a finger over his "trach" and croaked: "You cut my throat, put me in a coffin and tell me I'm the one who's crazy?"

A LIFETIME IN MEDICINE

Next to the Old Parkland stood the student nurses' quarters and classrooms. The annual infusion of fresh young girls brought an uplifting bloom to the old hospital. Nurses were all female then, many of them healthy, eager girls from large families who lived in small towns, farms and ranches. Usually there were one or two (three in a good year) who were achingly beautiful in their distinctive blue and white striped uniforms, starched white caps, white aprons, stockings and shoes. The mix of healthy young men and women in the jostle and bustle of strenuous, physical duties led to inevitable sexual tension. There would be the occasional firm breast pressed against one's arm or back. The work was too demanding and supervisors too numerous and vigilant for any carrying on during duty hours, save for perhaps the rare, furtive coupling down in the basement chart storage room or some dark closet, but there were ample opportunities for socializing among the singles at other times. Recently, one of my distinguished classmates told me how he and one of the truly spectacular OB nurses occasionally inhaled nitrous oxide (laughing gas) between deliveries. Once every a year or two there would be a hurry-up marriage, the nurse or student nurse beginning to show.

Because I was newly and very happily married, as well as ferociously focused on duty, I was able to elude these distractions.

On the other hand, my father, an unmarried intern at Parkland in the 1920s, apparently welcomed them. His reputation lingered long after his departure. One night at 2 or 3 a.m., I was on the elevator, a very slow, old elevator, with the night supervisor, a woman of about my father's age, whom I knew to be a Parkland veteran of many years. We rode in silence for a moment. Then:

"Dr. Roberts, is your father a doctor?"

"Yes, he is."

"Is his name the same as yours?"

"Yes."

"Did he intern at Parkland?"

"Yes, ma'am."

Whereupon Sadie Butler turned her head slightly to one side, touched her hand to her mouth, and snickered. Then the elevator stopped, and we parted.

The nursing students' graduation day included a ritual that would shock and awe our politically rectified generation. We ripped off their worn and faded candy stripes and aprons. Mostly, the undergraduate nurses did this, but we got into it as much as we could. The newly minted RN's clutched a few rags around slips or petticoats, laughing and blushing and then dashed for their quarters.

The Move

We moved everything from the Old Parkland to the New Parkland in a 24-hour period in the fall of 1954. In order to minimize transfers, we discharged every patient we could. It seemed to go remarkably well. That first night, I shared a room with my classmate, John Gunn, a rotating intern who was bound for a career in orthopedic surgery.

One patient's death may have been related to the move, a woman with severe diabetic ketoacidosis who went into shock and died. A vital datum-- the blood count -- was not reported until too late, and a critical anemia went undiagnosed and untreated.

My own recollections of old and new Parkland are blurred at times. I know we were at Old Parkland when my classmate Andy Gwynne, on duty in the ER, paged me to come see and admit a case of "bullous pemphigus." I found a dirty, destitute middle-aged man with many large blisters. On further questioning, we learned he was a vagrant who was living under one of the Trinity River viaducts. He and a couple of companions had consumed a quantity of cheap wine and had built a fire for warmth and to heat up food. Our patient had fallen into the fire, and his friends had doused him with some flammable liquid, probably alcohol. Fortunately, the burns were mainly second-degree, and he recovered.

The blistered vagrant was not the most gruesome sight I observed during my training. Far from it. Here are five of the worst memories that won't fade. Each occurred in the Emergency Room.

One night a policeman, looking quite grave, asked me to "pronounce" some fire victims. I followed him to his squad car. He opened the trunk. There were the completely charred – blackened – bodies of five small children. I don't know that this act by the policeman was actually required then or now. Perhaps he needed someone else to share the experience.

On another night – in my memories of the ER, it is always night – an old man was brought in with advanced and untreated cancer of the penis. Over the years, the cancer had completely eroded the penis and spread over the lower abdominal wall almost to the navel. The cancerous area was thickened, ulcerated, weeping -- and crawling with maggots. We should have been grateful for the maggots: these busy little creatures are still perhaps the most efficient way to clean and debride wounds of devitalized tissues, purulent matter and stench. A similar case involved a woman with untreated breast cancer. This I saw more than once. It was not all that rare in those days.

Another night, a body was brought in to be officially pronounced. A black woman had been asleep on the edge of a highway, her head resting on the highway's edge. A huge truck had run over her head, and the cranium was neatly severed as if by an ax, just above the ears. The base of the cranium was clean, like an empty bowl.

And then there was the suicide of my former stepfather, John Rodgers Moroney. He and my mother had been divorced for a few years. He was a brilliant, handsome and gifted man and a successful attorney. He was also a severe bipolar manic-depressive whose illness had grown progressively worse over the years. On the night of his death, he went alone to the ninth floor of the Santa Fe Building, where there was a radio station. Witnesses saw him calmly walk out the door to the surrounding parapet and climb over the wall. He jumped and apparently landed flat on his back, for his unmarked body was strangely flattened when it arrived at the ER. His expression was serene, the composure familiar to me. I confirmed his identity for the police.

Sometime later, I began to question whether I had actually seen all that I have just related. It was at a time that stories about false memories were coming out. But then I recalled that I had gone home and called my mother and brother, John, Jr. in Houston and told them what had happened.

Except for the burnt children and my stepfather's suicide, none of these encounters evoked much conscious emotion in me. Medical training equips us with psychological armor, and I had probably been already preconditioned by my childhood and my own father's example. All too often, doctors appear callous and flippant. Intern braggadocio is particularly annoying. And yet, as my story may attest, we become inured in order to have the resilience to confront, endure, persist and make sound medical decisions.

The great trick, of course, is never to lose our basic humanity. Not all doctors succeed at this. The good physician must be able to feel a bit of what the patient is feeling, while maintaining the distance necessary for objectivity. In the primary care specialties, where therapeutic relationships must be sustained over years or decades, this ability is indispensable. It is less so in other specialties, for example pathology, anesthesiology, radiology, intensive care – fields that require other skills and qualities.

During my senior year, I did some moonlighting at the old Gilbert and Roberts Clinic in Irving, Texas, then little more than a village of a few thousand people. The doctors there had some medical students and Interns to cover the clinic from 6 p.m. - 6 a.m. At 6 p.m., doctors and staff promptly departed, leaving us to handle whatever showed up. Most of the four or five of us who did this were not even M.D.'s yet. But we had completed our rotations in surgery, medicine, pediatrics, and OB-GYN. We were definitely practicing medicine without a license and with no medical liability insurance at all. But the clinic doctors needed help, the patients were grateful for the night clinic, and we needed the money.

The first part of the night usually wasn't too bad, mostly minor injuries and illnesses. Anyone needing hospitalization or urgent medical or surgical evaluation was sent to Methodist Hospital in Oak Cliff, where the doctors had admitting privileges, or to Parkland. At about 10 p.m., we locked the front door. After that, patients came to the back door, where they rang the bell. Night shifts could be scary, dramatic, and even dangerous. Some of the worst moments were during the polio epidemic. One night I unlocked the door to see a little boy of three or four, barely able to stand, his little legs collapsing under him. The anxious young parents told the story: headache, high fever, onset earlier that morning. I sent them straight to Parkland Hospital and asked about him the following day, learning that the child had died of bulbar polio.

Another night, a young pastor came in with similar symptoms, already struggling to swallow and breathe. He died at Parkland the next day. Sometimes the Irving police would bring in accident victims for evaluation. During my last night at the clinic, the police brought in a man with a head injury. I made a skull X-ray, which revealed a fracture. By this time, the patient was unconscious with one pupil dilated, both signs of life-threatening intracranial bleeding. I called Dr. Joe Roberts (not a relation), awakening him sometime after midnight. He told me to admit the patient to Methodist in his name and order some aspirin, that he would see the patient in the morning. This I did, making sure the admitting nurse knew it was a critical head injury.

I don't know what became of the patient. But the next day I called Joe Roberts and told him I wouldn't be moonlighting at his clinic anymore. I should make it clear that Joe Roberts was a fine surgeon, a good doctor, stalwart in his community and hospital for many years. He may well have awakened fully and decided to go to the hospital or called a neurosurgeon. Still, I'd had enough.

Wards

Hospital wards were segregated by race and sex: white male, white female, black male and black female. Each medical team was assigned to a ward of about two dozen beds, a dozen or so on each side of the room with a corridor down the middle and windows along the outside walls. The wards were on either side of a long connecting hallway. The ward team consisted of a resident, one or two Interns and a contingent of third-year students, typically four or five, plus a supervising faculty member and a town attending.

There were rooms with one or two beds for patients with contagious diseases and others who needed to be isolated.

Large wards – almost extinct today -- had a distinct sociology. Patients interacted with each other and with caregivers. Some visual privacy could be provided by simple screens, but mainly we were all out in the open, doctors, patients, nurses, and students. This created a shared experience. The resulting gemische depended on the condition and mood of the ward team and the quality of the interactions among them: the team members with each other, the team with the patients, and among the patients themselves.

It was not until later when I was in the Army serving as the sole physician in charge of a large, critically ill ward, that I truly appreciated ward dynamics. If morning and evening rounds went well and if my staff and I were congenial with the patients and one other, I would get a good night's sleep. If rounds were tense and the atmosphere was unpleasant, the opposite happened: the heart patients and ulcer patients suffered pain, the diabetics went out of control, and my phone rang and rang. There I learned for myself one of the most basic of lessons: to a huge extent, the doctor, along with the nurses and support team, is the medicine.

ALBERT D. ROBERTS, MD

Fatigue

The years from 1954, when I graduated, to 1975, when I left private practice to become an Associate Dean at UT Southwestern, are dominated by the memory of fatigue. One may read about it in medical journals, novels and personal histories of physicians, combat soldiers and young mothers, but never have I seen an account that conveys what I experienced in its full flower.

When you are young and eager, full of energy and zeal, you are unaware of fatigue for many hours. When it manifests itself, it may be disguised, denied and suppressed for a long time. For the first 12 to 18 hours or so, depending on the rigor of the shift, you don't feel tired. Then you are aware of being tired during the moments when you are not physically or mentally busy. Lying down for a minute, you fall asleep at once, but awaken quickly. Then, as the shift gets into the early morning hours with little or no rest, there may be an hour or two of fairly severe fatigue, mental and physical. I don't recall feeling mentally or physically impaired at such times; rather, I might ignore or delay a task that would have been quickly dispatched earlier in the shift. I became more economical and selective in order to preserve energy, or so I like to believe.

As the hours wear on, the fatigue gives way to a kind of resurrection, a physical anesthetization, and a sense, perhaps illusory, of heightened mental clarity and euphoria. I remember walking the long corridors and not feeling my feet touch the floor, or writing out my fifth or sixth admission automatically, without thinking. Sometimes I went to sleep while walking. Once I fell sound asleep at Thanksgiving dinner at the house of charitable friends.

There were epiphanies.

On the evening of Christmas Day, 1954, around 10 p.m., I remember writing up an admission, seated at the desk by the chart rack. I cradled my head in my arms and fell into a deep sleep instantly. Presently I became aware of a heavenly choir. I didn't know if I was awake or dreaming. I couldn't physically feel anything. Then down the long, darkened corridor came a slow procession of student nurses in their blue and white striped uniforms, starched white aprons and caps, caroling; the little candles held cupped in their hands softly lighted their faces. "O Holy Night," made ecstasy by beauty and exhaustion.

Other fatigue-related phenomena were more instructive than inspirational. I experienced sleep paralysis more than once, being awakened abruptly in the fourth stage of sleep, unable to move for several seconds. At such moments, I would be grateful for medical knowledge, able to know what was happening.

Looking back, I don't recall many errors that I can ascribe to fatigue. I made plenty of mistakes in a long career, but I attribute them to other reasons.

Learning, Teaching – And an Unorthodox Treatment

Our training in the '50s was remarkable for the paucity of teaching faculty and the intensity of the interaction. For a while only Dr. Seldin, Dr. Leonard Madison and Dr. Alvin Shapiro were full-time in the Department of Internal Medicine, bolstered by Dr. Ernest Muirhead from Pathology and Dr. Arthur Grollman, who had his own Department of Experimental Medicine (consisting of himself). For a brief time, in fact, Dr. Seldin had been the sole incumbent; that was before I went on the wards. As the '50s went along there came Dr. Carleton Chapman in Cardiology, Bill Miller in Pulmonology, A.I. Braude in Infectious Disease, Morris Ziff, Rheumatology; Eugene Frenkel in Hematology/Oncology. Still a tiny faculty by any standard, so they made teaching rounds nearly all year around. This close and frequent contact and the circumstances in which it occurred made for a learning experience of unparalleled intensity. Later, friends in medicine from the great established teaching centers would ask if we weren't somehow deprived, or wondered how any of us managed to turn out well. None of us ever felt this way, and our subsequent careers would bear this out. As such a large part of the House officers' experience involves one's fellow Interns, Residents and subspecialty fellows, I was remarkably fortunate, for the intern classes of '54 -'55 and '55 -'66 and later were remarkable. I have mentioned prominent members of my class, '54. The next year came Jean Wilson, Dan Foster, John Ribble, and Mack Perry. The following year came John Fortrand and Jack Barnett, each of whom has contributed meaningfully to medical research and education.

My distinction from those years, such as it is, is to have been Chief Resident for longer than anyone else has before or since. This came about because some of the senior Residents had been drafted or else fled elsewhere to escape from us aggressive young Turks. I was Dr. Seldin's third choice, actually. His favorite, Floyd Rector wisely declined and recommended me. Dr. Seldin chose Charlie Baxter instead. Charlie soon was drafted also. So in the spring of 1956, about two-thirds of the way through my third year (second year resident, after internship) I became the Chief Resident. My duties included arranging all the rotations, planning conferences, monitoring quality standards throughout the medicine service, and, not least, carrying on a tradition in our department by running the slide projector at conferences. I also did a lot of teaching of house staff and students. Because there were so few of us, I also assigned myself throughout the year to ward, emergency room and subspecialty rotations, taking my turn at night duty along with the others. Miraculously, I was also paid. There existed then a National Institutes of Health Extramural Fellowship Program intended to further the careers of promising, academically oriented Residents. It was a generous stipend for that time, about $500 a month. It enabled Diane to stop teaching and refocus on having children. This NIH Extramural Program (mine was in "diseases of metabolism") only lasted a short while, probably because so few of us fulfilled our early promise of real research and academic careers. I feel that I have repaid my debt by a lifetime of teaching, but have done very little research.

Being Chief was a role that I was comfortable with and carried out reasonably well, but there was the downside that I failed to develop any sustained research interest. It was easier and more fun to treat patients, teach and help organize the service. This would narrow my options early on, in effect defining my future career. In those days, there was no future in our department for anyone not driven to do research.

There were superb House officers. Jack Barnett and John Fortrand stand out as perhaps the best Interns I had when I was Chief. Jack became an expert in infectious disease and a famous alcoholic. Entering recovery, he was for many years Chief of Internal Medicine at Methodist Hospital in Dallas and prominent in physician recovery programs and in teaching students about addiction, along with sharing his vast general expertise. John Fortrand was Chief of Gastroenterology at UT Southwestern for many years before becoming Chief of Internal Medicine at Baylor University Medical Center. Throughout his long career, he has maintained a major research enterprise that included writing textbooks and articles.

Jack and I had one patient that I have waited a half century to tell about. All this time she has been in my mind: a black woman, in her

30s, dying of lupus. In appearance, a skeletal death camp survivor, miserable and wracked by pain and fever. She had the characteristic mouth ulcers, hair loss and skin rash, large, deeply pitted areas. Corticosteroids and antimalarials were the sole accepted treatment, and nothing was working. At about that time, an article appeared in the Archives of Internal Medicine by N.B. Kurnick (97:562, May 1956) entitled "A Rational Therapy of Systemic Lupus Erythematosus." Kurnick had previously published (Journal of Clinical Investigation, March 1953) that white blood cells inhibited the LE cell phenomenon. This clustering of white blood cells around globs of DNA was then the only diagnostic test for lupus, and Kurnick and others speculated that it was also a laboratory manifestation of the actual disease process. Kurnick had also noticed that leukemic white blood cells were better at blocking the LE cell phenomenon (in the lab) than normal white blood cells. The May 1956 article described 12 case histories of patients with advanced treatment-resistant lupus. The first ones were treated with injections of compatible blood from healthy volunteers, initially 30 milliliters intramuscularly three times a week. Several of the patients later received injections of WBCs only; this required only four or five cc's, and blood compatibility was not a requisite. The 12th patient received only a freeze-dried extract of white cells.

At least one patient (Case 5, page 572) received five milliliters of WBC from a leukemia patient. The results were reported as good in seven cases, doubtful in two and poor in two. Oddly, the 12th case, who was treated and retreated with "fractions of leukocytes...from bank blood" and seems to have done fairly well, is not counted in the summary. Kurnick's cases, like our one case, exhibited the full array of SLE manifestations: widespread inflammation of joints, sclerosal services (linings of heart, lung and peritoneum), skin, heart, kidneys and nervous system. And just like our case, the patients were not responding to orthodox treatment.

Thus it was that Jack and I elected to try "hemoinnoculation" on our patient. I was emboldened in part by the recollection that I personally had received hemoinnoculation therapy. The spring when I was 7, I was ill for a month with measles and complications, mainly an otitis media that would neither drain nor subside. My younger brother Bobby had recovered promptly, so our physician father drew a large syringe of blood from Bobby and stuck it in my behind. I soon recovered, but more credit may be due to my being the very first person to whom my father gave the new sulfonamide, Prontosil.

I went to Dr. Seldin and told him what we wanted to do, citing the Kurnick articles. He said to go ahead. None of this is in writing, of course (except in the long-gone patient's chart).

Next we found a donor, a source of WBCs. There was at that same time on the black female medicine ward an elderly woman with chronic lymphocytic leukemia. Her counts were in the 200,000 to 300,000 per milliliter range, so she was a rich source of WBCs. We drew her blood, centrifuged it, skimmed off the five milliliters or so of WBCs (the "buffy coat") and injected this into our patient intramuscularly, not IV. Kurnick said IM worked better. The patient improved dramatically and quickly. After about three injections, we discharged her to be followed in clinic. She was soon "lost to follow-up" so I don't anything of her subsequent course.

This adventure in informal experimental therapy occurred many decades before Institutional Review Boards (IRBs). Nothing of this sort could (or should) be attempted today. Such a departure from the strict regulations – not to mention ethics – of today would result in harsh penalties to the perpetrators and the individuals and institutions that sanctioned it.

Kurnick's discursive, anecdotal narratives and speculations are casual by today's standards and would never pass peer review. They might be acceptable as a letter to the editor.

As far as I am aware, this avenue of experimental treatment was not carried forward. And a subsequent review of the treatment of lupus (Annals of Internal Medicine, August 1956; (45, 163-184) by E.L. Dubois, then one of the most authoritative experts on the subject, mentioned Kurnick's treatment dismissively, saying it had been tried on one or two patients without effect. And that seems to have ended the story. Jack Barnett and I went on with our many tasks and responsibilities and did not try the treatment again.

Terminal Events

The last few months of my residency were memorable for several reasons. It was a happy time. We had a two-bedroom, two-story apartment, new and attractive. I was happy and secure in my role. We had two cars – a beautiful 1953 Studebaker Starlight Coupe and a 1954

Pontiac Chieftain two-door hardtop on loan from Diane's parents. Our son David Truett was born on March 10, 1957 and we were delighted, and very relieved to have a perfectly formed healthy baby boy, though he was quite irritable for a few months.

A couple of weeks after Diane and Truett came home from the hospital the great tornado of 1957 struck, April 6th.

It was in the afternoon. I had been on duty the day and night before, in the ER. The weather had been ominous all day – boiling greenish-blue storm clouds surging southwest to northeast as Canadian and Gulf systems collided all along a diagonal across Texas and into Arkansas and Oklahoma and beyond. I was standing upstairs in the bathroom when I saw it, just a couple of miles south of our apartment, a huge, black funnel spinning violently and moving erratically northwest. It came fairly close to Parkland, crossing Harry Hines Boulevard at Record Crossing, before dissipating. I could see objects falling out of the funnel. I went to the apartment courtyard, sirens and alarms making a cacophony – and saw many little vortices nearby and just overhead and Diane standing anxiously in the doorway, holding our infant son.

Then I went back to work. We had just, within the previous couple of weeks, performed a detailed disaster drill at Parkland. It was the era of fear of atomic holocaust. All the Parkland doctors had an assigned role. Mine was medical consultant to the surgical trauma ward. We wore armbands for identification. Each unit was fully prepared and manned with efficient medical and surgical teams. In the event, there was not a great deal to do. There were six or eight deaths and 100 or so injuries, but they did not all come to Parkland. It was not very different from a busy Saturday night; at least not once you got inside the hospital. Getting there was the problem. All the streets were crammed with thrill seekers. Ambulances couldn't get through. I parked about a mile from the hospital, about halfway from our apartment, and trotted to my station.

The great thing about the tornado was that it heralded the end of the seven-year drought. The spring and summer were among the coolest and wettest ever. But Diane, Truett and I missed most of that. Starting July 1, 1957, I was in the Army of the United States.

Chapter 4

05407582

That is my number. While the general military draft had ended after the Korean War, the doctor draft continued, with one brief interruption around 1960, until after the Vietnam War. All fledgling Army doctors were required to attend a six-week indoctrination course at Fort Sam Houston in San Antonio. We went to class morning and afternoon and learned the rudiments of military medicine. I remember almost nothing of that, but I liked the course in the proper use of the field compass and topographic map.

We went into the field for an overnight bivouac experience at Camp Bullis, which was notorious for "Bullis Fever," a tick-borne disease similar to typhus that was endemic there. We were impressed as we observed while troops erected a Mobile Army Surgical Hospital (MASH) in a few minutes. Inside the tent, a drill was staged to simulate combat conditions. Anesthetized goats that had been shot in the thigh were placed on the operating tables, and we repaired the wounds.

"What becomes of the goats?" someone asked.

"Cabrito," another answered.

No cabrito for us. We dined on cold K-rations, which aren't too bad if you're really hungry.

We heard some lectures in the afternoon and fired 45-caliber pistols and carbines. That night, we gamely crawled perhaps a hundred yards or so over hard, stony ground and under barbed wire, while allegedly live machine gunfire whizzed overhead.

Our instructors, veteran sergeants with many hash marks on their sleeves, somberly told us of the naïve soldier who jumped up when the firing started and was shot through. True or not, every class heard the story in those years, and it did, indeed, motivate us to keep our heads down.

Those were years when things military were not much admired. Drafted doctors typically reacted with rancor, or at best, grudging resignation, to this intrusion on their lives and career plans.

I was one of the few who liked the Army. At times, I loved it. First, there was Fort Sam Houston, hallowed ground and home to many generations of soldiers dating from the mid-19th century to the end of the 20th century. From the red brick barracks and duplex officers' quarters to the grand parade ground, Reveille in the morning, and Retreat at sundown, I found it all rich and satisfying. The largest of the red brick homes, for the senior officers and the Commandant, were in a line along one side of the parade ground. Back then, the current occupant's name was displayed on a small sign. Beside it was a bronze plaque commemorating some famous former occupant: Arthur McArthur, John J. Pershing, Dwight Eisenhower, and Robert E. Lee.

The new, young (and a few not so young) military doctors were quartered in large enlisted men's barracks with high-ceilinged rooms, rows of metal cots and footlockers and no air conditioning in the south Texas August. I don't recall that bothering me. We were all acclimatized, and the rooms were large and well ventilated. Each morning we mustered in the quadrangle. A brass band on the balcony across the quadrangle from the formation played marches, often Colonel Bogey's March, as we filed off to our morning classes. We ate sturdy army food in a large mess hall. Not as good as home cooking, but better than Parkland. The rule was, "take all you want, eat all you take."

It was no bad thing, being a 27-year-old captain in the Army Medical Corps and marching off to class with a brass band playing.

During my six weeks there, I read Thucydides' account of the Peloponnesian Wars and reread the Battle of Borodino in War and Peace. Weekends, I drove or flew Trans-Texas Airlines, affectionately known as "Treetop Airlines," low-flying old DC-3 Gooney Birds without air conditioning, home to Dallas to be with Diane and our infant son.

That six-week period was the first completely carefree time I'd had since my summers as a camper, counselor or lifeguard. Diane, on the other hand, had been left alone five days a week to care for our four-month-old son. Truett was beautiful, blessedly healthy and adorable, except when colicky or crying, as he frequently was. She never complained.

There was some sort of graduation ceremony. Diane came down on the train, her first respite from her new responsibilities. We dined with friends at Jack's, a famous steakhouse, and the next day Captain and Mrs. Albert D. Roberts, Jr., U.S. Army, MC, returned to Dallas. We closed out the apartment there on Bordeaux, traded the beautiful 1953 Studebaker Starlight Coupe for a sturdy utilitarian '57 Ford Ranch Wagon with two doors, huge V8, three-speed column shift and rudimentary air conditioning. I meticulously arranged our luggage in the capacious aft compartment.

Setting off on our journey to a new and very different life, we stopped off to say good-bye to the Truetts. Mamie had one of her trademark conniptions. Standing there in the driveway, bidding our farewells, Mamie abruptly demanded that I totally reconfigure the luggage that I had so carefully arranged; I had done it all wrong. I demurred, gently, I hope. On the way out of town, I called in a tranquilizer prescription for Mamie, a parting gesture on my part. Mamie and Fred were always and from the beginning extremely kind and generous to me, despite well-founded misgivings, and to us, but this little scene dramatized the positive benefits of our young family getting away on its own for a couple of years.

For our four-month-old Truett, we arranged a platform pen/bed that filled the back seat. He could roll around a bit and sleep as much as he wanted. His former irritability and frequent crying miraculously disappeared, and he slept most of the way to Chattanooga, where we visited my father and his third wife Lora, who were renting a stone cottage high up on Signal Mountain. The cottage was called "The Pot-o-Gold House" after the fey decoration at the base of the mailbox. Nestled among tall, fragrant pines, it perched serenely there, its ample stone terrace overlooking a bend in the Tennessee River and its vast valley far below.

Diane and I had visited there twice before, once by train and once by car, and we returned twice more during my two years in the Army. It was the last good period in Pop and Lora's life together and the only time we were all really comfortable. That seven or eight years they had there on Signal Mountain was a plateau in his long and tragic deterioration.

A LIFETIME IN MEDICINE

They had fled Fort Worth abruptly in 1949, with Pop beset by tort lawyers, creditors and the IRS. It was a shocking reversal of fortune brought on by mental illness. He had returned from WWII service in 1946, age 44, primed for a brilliant career in plastic surgery.

During the Great Depression, he had started out as a general practitioner in Fort Worth after a less-than-complete internship at Parkland Hospital in Dallas. He practiced alone and did reasonably well using his skill, enterprise and intelligence. He gradually branched out into general surgery. In the mid-1930s, he became fascinated with plastic surgery. I remember him sitting in the living room, reading and modeling clay noses and ears long into the night.

He arranged preceptorships with two of the most famous plastic surgeons of the day. The first was the great Gustave Offrich of New York. The second was in San Francisco. I've forgotten his name, but it was one of the grand events of childhood for Bobby and me. Pop bought a trailer, took me out of the first grade in the fall of 1936, and off we went across prairie, desert and mountains to California.

At that time, he was married to Lucille Gordon, whom he had married not long after he and mother divorced. Mother had a severe depression after Bobby was born in November of 1931, and after months of hospitalization, she returned to her family in Ft Worth. Pop retained custody, and we lived with him and Lucille until 1941. Our Roberts half-brother, George, was born Christmas Eve, 1938. Lucille decamped abruptly with George in December of 1940. Pop enlisted in the Army Medical Corps in 1941, and Bobby and I spent the rest of our childhood in Dallas with our mother and her new husband, John R. Moroney, general counsel and partner in Interstate Theaters.

After induction at the Carlisle Barracks in Pennsylvania and a brief time in Victoria, Texas, Pop was assigned to the Army Air Corps Strategic Air Command (SAC) hospital in San Antonio, where he soon became chief of the Burn Unit. The burned airmen who survived to arrive in San Antonio or who did not die shortly afterward, as many did, required a great deal of plastic surgery. My father acquired great skill with skin grafts and reconstructive surgery. He also took justifiable pride in his tendon repairs, delicate work that only a few master.

Pop and Lora were married not long after his enlistment. He had begun an affair with her months before when she was married to one of his golfing buddies. The affair was Lucille's main reason for fleeing.

Lora, from Cleburne, Texas, was attractive, smart and completely devoted to my father. It was the best of his three marriages.

So the future was bright for the still-young surgeon returning from the war, his skills burnished by fire, so to speak.

It did not last long. His amphetamine use had probably started in the Army, where it was common practice in wartime. As his initially successful post-war practice became busier, his abuse became heavier. Amphetamines in the morning and barbiturates at night led to an elaborate paranoid psychosis. His work deteriorated. There were bad results and patients sued. His debts accumulated. He never paid his income tax.

One day, he and Lora just disappeared. But first, he dispatched Bobby, who was living with them and attending Texas Christian University, to the University of Texas with $100 in his pocket and abandoned him. Then he and Lora packed up and drove off in the blue 1946 Lincoln Continental convertible with $50,000 cash (Bobby says it was $250,000) and a .38-caliber revolver in the glove compartment.

They went west, staying a few weeks at a time in inexpensive motels and obscure inns and resorts. He recovered from his psychosis and addiction. I had only one contact with them during this interval. Pop touched down in Dallas just long enough to have a hemorrhoidectomy performed at Baylor hospital by his classmate, Jack Kerr.

After two years of this wandering, he got a job as the plant physician at the DuPont plant in Chattanooga, and that's how we all got together.

Eventually, the Chattanooga interlude also fell apart, and the downward spiral resumed. They lived for a while in Austin, then Corpus Christi, and finally Houston, to be near the Veterans Hospital as his lung disease worsened. He had been a three-pack-a-day smoker for over 40 years. They lived mainly on the military service disability payments that Lora had pursued, service-connected because his lung problems had begun in the Army. He died shortly after his 70th birthday in 1972. Lora died with Alzheimer's disease a few years later.

I loved and admired my father. He was gifted with a keen and critical intelligence, as well as remarkable physical skills. He could tie square knots with his left hand in his pants pocket. His illness and

A LIFETIME IN MEDICINE

decline were terrible to witness. I had to distance myself emotionally in order to get on with my own life, but I am grateful for the childhood years in Fort Worth and the long talks on the terrace up on Signal Mountain.

We arrived at Fort Dix, New Jersey, August 1957, at the start of a flu epidemic. 1957 was a bad pandemic year. Over a couple of weeks, all three of us had it, even I, who had begun to think myself unassailable by contagion, having not had even a cold in several years. Fortunately, none of us was very sick; it just added to the discomfort of being crammed into a single room in the Bachelor Officers Quarters until proper housing could be found.

Soon we were comfortable in our new two-story, two-bedroom unit in Wherry Housing apartments, brick veneer multiple dwelling buildings, each with a large commons in front and parking behind. For the lucky wives there was a huge laundry facility in a close-by brick building and clotheslines for drying the wash. Soon our own furniture arrived, and we settled in for our military experience.

Fort Dix sprawls over a large part of central New Jersey. It is flat country, the original pine and hardwood forests long gone, except for an odd anachronistic backwater not far from Fort Dix called "the Pineys." Fort Dix had been Camp Dix in World War I, when it was the major facility for assembling troops who were shipping off to France. We have something of a family history there. My stepfather, John R. Moroney, a 19-year-old Second Lieutenant, was there when the war ended in November 1918. He recalled his troop train arriving at the Dix Station and seeing the platform stacked high with the plain, pine coffins of young soldiers, victims of the great influenza pandemic of 1918-1919. Diane's father, Fred Truett, also a teenage shavetail, born in 1899, as was John Moroney, was stationed in Nashville and had orders in hand to proceed to Dix when the war ended.

Assigned to the Army Air Corps Medical Corps, the Army first sent Pop for indoctrination to the Carlisle Barracks in Pennsylvania, not far from Fort Dix. He extolled Bookbinder's Restaurant to Diane and me when our turn came. We found it and Philadelphia little changed in the 15 years since Pop had eaten and drunk there.

The hospital was a general hospital with more than 1,200 beds and a complete staff, all Army except for civilian secretaries and some technical support, engineers, technicians and skilled laborers. It was a

World War II leftover, all one floor, all wooden, mostly plywood, the outside painted that same flat pale yellow as all such buildings from that era. The corridors seemed about a half-mile long. But it had nearly everything that a big municipal hospital required and functioned much the same, although with a somewhat different clientele. Fort Dix was a basic training camp; up to 40,000 recruits were there at any given time. We also served another population of approximately 60,000 retired military personnel and their families, as well as families of active military personnel in the area, mainly central and southern New Jersey.

In addition, we served McGuire Air Force Base, headquarters of the Northeastern Fighter Command as well as the Military Air Transport Service (MATS). Back then, the Air Force had only flight surgeons, generally people with the equivalent of a rotating internship and a bit of additional ENT and ophthalmology training. They had no specialists and no hospitals, only outpatient clinics and small infirmaries in remote areas. Thus they utilized Army or Navy resources for specialty and hospital care. There were also referrals from the other military installations scattered about New Jersey such as Fort Belvoir and the Naval Air Station at Lakehurst. This situation augured a rich medical experience.

However, my first few days in the medicine service were far from sanguine.

To begin with, there was Colonel Ed Cleave, the soon-to-retire Chief of the Medicine Service. I marched into his office, stood at attention, saluted smartly, and said, "Captain Albert D. Roberts reporting for duty, sir."

Behind the desk slumped a thin, dispirited, sallow man with sunken dark eyes and dark hair, in rumpled service khaki. He looked me over, his expression bemused and disinterested.

"At ease," he responded sardonically, and then he hauled his emaciated body almost erect, shuffled wordlessly to the nearby sink, and urinated.

Something closer to my expectations occurred when I presented myself to the hospital Commandant, a wispy little man and a courteous Southerner, who, like Colonel Cleave, was soon to retire. The Commandant and his wife had lived extensively in the Orient and had collected many beautiful objects. Diane and I were invited to tea. The Commandant's wife gave Diane the official manual on the proper etiquette and deportment for officers' wives: hats, gloves, courtesy calls, bridge parties, teas and so on. My favorite etiquette tidbit was "When shopping with your husband, you must always carry the parcels in case he needs to salute."

There were six of us new arrivals, including Colonel Cleave's replacement, Lieutenant Colonel Ray Blohm, who was a fine doctor and an excellent officer. Ray and his wife Betty became friends to all of us. One of the doctors we replaced was Gerald Weissman, who became a famous rheumatologist, author and editor. He edited Hospital Practice, for many years the best of the "throwaway" journals, modeled after Scientific American. Dr. Weissman and I had a brief, cordial exchange some years later following a piece he did reminiscing about his two years at Fort Dix.

The incoming group included Dick and Nelda Romig from California and Dave and Nancy Glassner from Wisconsin. We all had young children and became not only good friends but also a much-needed mutual support group. Everybody's favorite pediatrician was Stan Rosenthal from Florida. He and his wife, Zelda, were also good friends.

The first week or so after our arrival, I was bidden to attend an official staffing procedure convened to address whether to medically discharge a young recruit with an enigmatic illness. There he sat, on a straight-backed cane bottom chair, encircled by perplexed doctors. The problem was that he could not perform the activities required of recruits due to weakness, fatigue and easy injuries. And yet there was nothing obviously wrong with him. He'd had all the tests anyone could think of, some of them two or three times. In fact, he had just returned from Walter Reed with a thick chart and no diagnosis.

The soldier had some odd-looking scars. On impulse I rose from my chair, stepped over by him, grasped his cheek firmly and pulled the skin easily two inches out, demonstrating the classical finding of cutis hyperelastica.

"An obvious case of Ehlers-Danlos Syndrome," I announced.

So the soldier got his medical discharge, and I got two weeks' assignment to a battalion aid station – Colonel Cleave's parting gift to me, something like in baseball player being sent to the minors, as a reward for my star turn.

On return from exile, I was assigned to the critically ill medical ward. So began perhaps the most challenging, exciting and rewarding 20 months of my entire medical career. Normally everyone rotated to a different service every couple of months. Not I. I loved the critical ward, and everyone else seemed intimidated by it, so Colonel Blohm let me keep it for the rest of my term of service.

Most mornings I walked the few blocks from our apartment to the hospital, beginning each day with morning ward rounds. Two nurses, a corpsman and I visited each patient in turn, chart rack in tow, beginning with the new admissions and the sickest patients. The night nurse would give a brief report; I would review each chart at the bedside, ask the patient a few questions, do whatever physical exam was called for, offer encouragement and give the nurses my orders for the day. There were about 40 beds in the open ward, plus two or three private rooms for the sickest patients or those requiring isolation. The beds were usually all occupied. Typically, there would be three or four very ill patients. Thus, my ward team could serve over 40 patients in an hour or two. Nothing of the sort is possible nowadays with patients all in private or semi-private rooms. On an open ward, a nurse and a corpsman could effectively manage 40 or 50 patients. What has been gained in privacy has been at a cost and not just expense and lost efficiency. There was also the open-ward social dynamic, the spontaneous natural support groups and camaraderie, and the humor – sometimes grim. Occasionally a negative clique would form, made up of one or two hostile "jailhouse lawyers" and a couple of adherents. You could immediately feel the atmosphere sour with complaints, demands, inappropriate symptoms, and sarcasm. Once recognized, these groups were easily dealt with, merely broken up by transfers to another service or to a far corner of the ward.

The ward system still prevails in the military, where efficiency takes priority.

After ward rounds there were consulting rounds. We had four consultants, all academically oriented internists from Philadelphia. Three were men of moderate attainments, not especially helpful themselves, though the case presentations often stimulated useful discussions. The fourth, Dr. Norman Lerner was as gifted a bedside teacher as any I encountered throughout my training and an excellent model for a young, academically oriented physician.

I liked to remember Dr. Lerner's example when a dozen or so years later, I was the visiting consultant to the Fort Wolters General Hospital in Mineral Wells, Texas.

A LIFETIME IN MEDICINE

A second consultant I remember mainly for his self-presentation. A well-regarded gastroenterologist well into his 60s, he drove out from Philadelphia in a 1950`s, short wheel base, razor-edge Bentley, two-tone black over gray. He wore meticulously aged three-piece gray suits. His manner was dignified, courtly, kind and sympathetic. I don't remember learning a lot from Dr. Wirtz, but he certainly fulfilled my expectation of how a big-time Philadelphia specialist should appear and comport himself.

Afternoons were spent in the outpatient clinic. This comprised six or eight individual office-cum-examining rooms in the same wing as the Internal Medicine administrative offices and support staff. Typically, I would see eight to twelve patients in an afternoon, more than half retired military families, but also active military, consultations from McGuire Air Force Base, and transients. I learned a good bit from these patients.

One I remember was a retired colonel in his 60s who had frequent spells of confusion, some lasting up to several hours. Otherwise, he was all right, an average retired officer of that generation – quiet and prematurely aged by hard service in World War II. The physical exam provided one critical clue: the edge of a small, hard, nodular liver could just be palpated with deep inspiration. There was no spleen palpable, and no jaundice or other signs of liver disease. Routine laboratory tests were normal.

On questioning, it developed that these spells tended to follow a high-protein meal. After eating a steak, the colonel experienced hours of somnolence and confusion. I suspected ammonia intoxication. Ammonia forms in the colon by the action of normal bacteria on urea; urea is a principal breakdown product of protein. Normally the ammonia is absorbed from the colon into the portal vein and transported to the liver, where the Krebs urea cycle metabolizes it. But the cirrhotic liver partially blocks the portal vein, diverting blood into the general circulation. Ammonia can then penetrate the brain with calamitous consequences.

A blood test for ammonia was not available, and his liver function tests fell almost within normal limits. My clues were the small, hard liver, plus his story. The colonel had been the officer responsible for military transport through the port of Antwerp. Tons of material came off the ships, onto land transport, through the city and on to many destinations. He worked around the clock, catching naps or a few hours' sleep when he could. He had no regular meals; his fuel was alcohol. Never drunk, he told me – and his record was unblemished – he just ran mainly on alcohol for many months. When it was over, he was left with a small, hard liver, some very good ribbons to wear and an acquired intolerance to protein.

I put him on a low-protein diet plus a low dose of Neomycin to discourage the bacteria. As long as he kept to this regimen, he had no spells. The received wisdom in those days was that antibacterial treatment was impractical and dangerous because huge doses were required in order to sterilize the gut. What my patient demonstrated was that killing off the normal flora wasn't necessary. All that is required is to deplete or debilitate the germs (make them sick) using, say, two grams per day of Neomycin instead of the recommended nine or 10 grams. Nowadays we know that maintaining rapid transit through the colon by means of laxation and avoiding protein loads is usually sufficient.

I can't forbear to note that this diagnosis and successful treatment strategy came about decades before sophisticated imaging studies and complex biochemical testing, by means of a careful history, meticulous physical exam and a therapeutic trial. The few tests available were nondiagnostic. Cost to the taxpayer: a piece of my small salary and a nanofraction of overhead.

The Critically Ill Ward

Many of the young trainees were desperately ill. This was not due to lack of surveillance in the field. There were effective procedures in place to identify and quickly transport sick soldiers. Rather it was because the young men sometimes would attempt to deny and conceal illness to avoid having to start over in basic training. If you dropped out of training for more than 72 hours, you were "recycled." The Medical Corps was highly sensitive to the need for early recognition and prompt treatment of ill soldiers. There had been two deaths from meningococcal infections and two congressional investigations in the two years prior to my arrival. But the problem remained that not a few young men would risk death before recycling.

I don't mean that the terrible illnesses I saw were all due to deliberate delays in getting medical treatment. In fact, most either had sought help appropriately or were quickly picked up by alert noncoms

A LIFETIME IN MEDICINE

and officers in the field. The Army medicine that I saw was highly professional, from the battalion aid station to the great general hospitals like Walter Reed.

Patients' stories best illustrate the variety and intensity of my medical experience during 20 months on the Critically Ill Ward.

Gary, about 20, lay on the examining table where the corpsmen had just placed him, paralyzed. He could not move his arms or legs, his breathing was shallow, and his voice weak with the characteristic flat nasal tone that indicated paralysis of the muscles of phonation. As I examined him, his breathing simply stopped. There was nothing like a modern respirator, only some oxygen, which we started. We got someone from Anesthesia to "bag" him – a facemask with a manually compressed balloon – but obviously, this was not a long-term solution. I asked if there were an iron lung somewhere. Blank responses. Then someone, I think it was Millie Distasi, the sainted Internal Medicine Office Manager, who recalled an old Drinker Respirator, the original iron lung, back in the warehouse, unused since the end of polio a few years before. This apparatus was located, quickly cleaned and found to be operative. This paleotechnic device was basically a large metal cylinder, about seven feet long and two feet in diameter, with a diaphragm at one end. At the other, an aperture provided an airtight seal around the patient's neck so that only the head protruded from the iron cylinder. The diaphragm was attached to an electric motor, rhythmically evacuating air from the airtight cylinder and, by vacuum, drawing it into the patient's lungs.

Prolonged respirator care required that the patient have a tracheostomy, and when Gary's condition did not improve after a few days, a surgeon was summoned and the procedure hurriedly performed. Calamitously, it was found to be too low in the neck and the airtight collar could not be fitted below the tracheostomy. Thus it was useless. Unless we could do something quickly, the patient would soon die.

Something could be done. This twelve hundred-bed Army hospital had a single Bennett intermittent positive pressure breathing (IPPB) machine, and it had tracheostomy attachments. I hooked Gary to the IPPB machine, his trach and his lifeline safely just barely inside the collar, his upper neck and head outside, supine. His eyes remained open, watching, and motionless.

There he remained for a month, totally paralyzed, fully conscious. He could not even blink. The nurses put patches on his eyes for him to sleep. The Drinker and the Bennett filled his lungs with air and kept him alive.

I was in charge of the ward where all this played out, and was the only physician who had experience (or would confess that he had) with polio and Drinkers. I was in effect on-call for Gary 24 hours a day for as long as he was there. He did not have poliomyelitis: he had the Guillain-Barré syndrome, an autoimmune disorder attacking the motor neurons of the nervous system. The spinal fluid was diagnostic: elevated protein, very few white blood cells. The disease may follow certain kinds of acute infections, and, as contagion is a universal accompaniment of the military experience, is something to be anticipated in the crowding and rigors of basic training. It was relatively common in my time at Dix. I believe I saw about six cases in all. All but Gary recovered, as do most, usually completely.

One afternoon while I was seeing patients in the clinic, a ferocious thunderstorm suddenly crashed around the hospital. Power had been disrupted and all the lights went out. I was transfixed, my mind blank with an unknown dread for a second or two, and suddenly it hit me: the iron lung! I ran as hard as I could the 25 or 30 yards from the clinic, across the hall and pell-mell into the ward, finding the nurses and corpsman dumbfounded and horrified, but the flexible diaphragm at the "breathing" end of the respirator had a big lever just for this purpose. Drinker had anticipated power failure! I grabbed the lever, and we took turns mechanically breathing Gary until power was restored, 15 or 20 long minutes.

Gary's mother, aunt and uncle had come from Manhattan, and they hovered close by. They were apparently influential people. When it became clear that Gary was not recovering, they were able to help us arrange his transfer by air ambulance to Walter Reed Army Hospital in Washington, D.C. They also tried to have me transferred along with him, but that didn't work. It was no use. Gary died at Walter Reed two or three weeks later.

The sickest person I saw who actually recovered was a good-looking 20-year-old recruit from Scarsdale, N.Y., where his father was a dentist. He was very ill on admission, blood pressure very low and pulse just palpable in the wrists. He lay supine, too weak to sit, covered with purple blotches and red spots, "petechiae," the characteristic features of acute meningococcemia. In addition, there were some ominous findings not characteristic of meningococcemia. His neck veins were bulging, and the cardiac examination disclosed that the normal muscular thrust of the left ventricle against the chest wall was absent. Instead, there was a faint, diffuse quiver. Percussion could not outline the borders of the heart. An X-ray revealed that the heart, so swollen it resembled a huge, flabby water bottle, filled the chest. The critical question was whether it was a giant pericardial effusion or myocarditis. If effusion, it was vital to draw off the fluid, a risky procedure in such a situation, but life-saving. If infection of the heart muscle, then nothing could be done but general supportive majors such oxygen and careful fluid therapy and hope that the antibiotics would do their work in time. We determined to try to remove fluid, performing a pericardiocentesis, a procedure I had done only once in the Parkland ER. Lieutenant Colonel Blohm, the Chief of Service, tried it there on the ward. A little local anesthetic, some reassuring words, then in went the needle. And out came blood; the needle was inside the heart, no fluid from the pericardial sac, no instant, decisive relief. Dick lay there, almost motionless, his sick heart barely pumping enough blood to sustain his vital organs. Then, after four or five very anxious days, he began to improve. Ultimately, he recovered completely.

This story has a coda. About 20 years later, a husband and wife who were patients of mine found themselves seated at dinner on a transatlantic voyage with a dentist from Scarsdale and his wife. Learning my patients were from Dallas, the dentist asked if by chance they knew a Dr. Roberts. From her purse, the Dallas wife produced a prescription medication with my name on the label.

There were to be in all 28 cases of meningococcal infections admitted to my service. They were about equally divided between those with meningococcemia manifested by skin rash and shock; those with meningitis, presenting with severe headache, altered consciousness and a stiff neck; and those who had both. There was even one case of mild, chronic meningococcemia.

The patient was a soldier who had just flown in from Germany. He asked to be seen for mild aching and malaise, thinking he might be coming down with the flu. And so he might, except for the lack of any respiratory signs or symptoms and for the eloquent little punctate skin hemorrhages – the telltale petechial rash – just a few, mainly clustered around the ankles. He was skeptical when I insisted on hospitalizing him, but sure enough, within 24 hours his blood cultures were growing out neisseria meningitides. He was never very ill and might well have recovered without treatment, but he likely would have exposed others, perhaps many others.

Another young man whom I remember particularly well, also a basic trainee, had purpura fulminans, the most serious form of meningococcemia. At its worst, it can cause a particularly nasty peripheral gangrene of the fingers, toes, nose, penis, sometimes leading to amputation, and often to death. This young man had purple palms and soles, almost black. Even today, this form of the disease is usually fatal, but this soldier recovered. We treated him with sulfonamide and penicillin, plus a corticosteroid, hydrocortisone or prednisone. This was my usual therapeutic strategy. As he recovered, the skin of his palms and soles sloughed off, leaving a new layer of tender, sensitive "baby" skin and, for this man, a very serious complication: hyperhydrosis, or extreme sweating. Before military service, he was in the hotel business, which required a great deal of greeting and handshaking. Wherever he walked, he left wet footprints, and when he wore shoes, they filled with fluid. Shaking his hand was like grabbing a full sponge; your own hand came away dripping wet. I don't know whether this condition persisted. He soon received his medical discharge from the Army.

All 28 cases of meningococcal infection recovered. I take some credit for this; my management was quick and decisive. In one or two cases, I may have been primarily responsible for successful outcomes. On two occasions, I re-examined spinal fluid samples that the lab tech and the pathologist had both reported as negative and found the presence of meningococci.

For this skill I was indebted to Dr. A.I. (Abe) Braude, Chief of Infectious Disease at Southwestern and Parkland, who required his Residents to begin each day by looking down the microscope at every one of the previous day's and night's specimens.

I have mentioned that we had a solitary Bennett IPPB breathing device. This was not "GI," or regulation government issue. We acquired ours because of a chance encounter. One afternoon walking along on one of the long hospital corridors, I met a very elderly couple, a wife pushing her husband in his wheelchair. They were lost and tired, and I helped them get to their car. A few days later, our Internal Medicine Chief, Dr. Blohm, summoned me to his office and showed me a letter from the man whom I had assisted, copied to the hospital Commandant, expressing gratitude and asking if there was anything I needed that the hospital lacked. It turned out that this man was the highest ranking retired U.S. Army Medical Officer, a former Surgeon General of the Army. I requested the Bennett machine, and in a few weeks one arrived.

The Bennett machine enabled us to keep our Guillain-Barré patient, Gary, alive until he could be transferred to Walter Reed Hospital. The Bennett and I unquestionably saved another soldier's life. I was urgently summoned to the orthopedic ward in consultation. There I found a man in grave respiratory distress from a flail chest sustained in a car wreck. The impact against the steering wheel had separated his ribs from his breastbone so that when he attempted to inhale, his chest caved in, and when he tried to exhale, it flailed outward. He was moving no air, despite tremendous effort. He had only his diaphragm to work with, and the flail chest rendered diaphragmatic excursions ineffectual. Despite a rate of 30 or 40 breaths per minute, he was cyanotic – blue all over – and tiring fast. The surgeons had immobilized his chest by inserting sharp forceps into the skin over the breastbone and attaching them to a fixed frame over the bed (rather like a Lakota initiation, but more therapeutic). This helped, but did not enable enough air exchange. I ran the quarter mile or so back to my ward, grabbed the Bennett machine, and ran with it back to the orthopedic ward, where I attached it to the patient. The soldier pinked right up, his panicky efforts subsided, and he survived.

Today he would be in a modern intensive care unit, attended by a team of lung specialists, respiratory technicians and RNs. A half-century ago, it was one primitive breathing machine and one young internist who knew how to use it in a 1,200-bed hospital. I remember many cases. Some haunt me, and some make me smile. There was a teenage Latin American boy, dwarfed by asthma and emphysema. His name was Asrubo, and his father was career Army. His mother worked, so he had responsibility for a bunch of younger siblings, while trying to stay in school and fighting for nearly every breath. Possibly he had alpha chymotrypsin deficiency or perhaps cystic fibrosis. He was all barrel chest, little spidery arms and legs, and he was cheerful all the time. I never saw him frown. He had never been on a cortisone preparation. I started him on prednisone, and he improved dramatically, even experiencing a growth spurt.

I also recall a recruit who had the worst Stevens-Johnson syndrome I've ever seen – skin covered with cat's eye lesions, all mucous membranes painfully ulcerated around his mouth, throat, nose and eyes. He couldn't swallow anything but liquids, and that hurt too. As recovery began at about the end of the first week (blessed prednisone again!), he coughed up a complete cast of his tracheobronchial tree, the fibrin, mucous and inflammatory debris displaced by new respiratory epithelium. This is something you read about in old texts. How many doctors alive today have seen this?

Then there was the 18-year-old inductee with juvenile diabetes who had joined the Army to "make a man of myself" and who had thrown away his insulin. In a few days, he was in deep diabetic ketoacidosis complicated by a ferocious pneumococcal pansinusitis, all sinuses packed with thick, creamy pus. He barely survived. Insulin, penicillin, lots of IV fluids – and youth – pulled him through. Then we sent him back home to his parents.

Sometimes, when the great respiratory disease epidemics, influenza, adenovirus, swept through, all of the 1,200 beds would be occupied. We would walk through these wards, hundreds of sick men (and women too, there was a female medicine ward for Army personnel and Army families) to try to pick out the ones who were seriously ill, the ones who had high fever, respiratory distress or just looked really sick. Inevitably, there were some cases of severe pneumonia, including staphylococcal pneumonia. One such patient was admitted to my ward in the middle of the night and died before I came back on duty in the morning.

Then there were the old sergeants, gray veterans of the wars, serving out their time until retirement. I saw several horrific cases of delirium tremens, horrible hallucinations, and body temperatures to 109, violent shaking all over. They were all right, performing their familiar, often simple and repetitive, jobs, as long as they had regular access to liquor. If they fell ill and had to be admitted to the hospital and deprived of their daily ration, the DT's would come on. Sometimes one would beg me to give him some alcohol to prevent or mitigate the dreaded withdrawal syndrome. I would refuse, little prig that I was, and I have always regretted that.

How I Got my Presidential Citation

The internists took Medical Officer of the Day (M.O.D.) emergency call in rotation. This duty entailed spending the night in the hospital emergency room. After 6 p.m., patients would come in from the Fort Dix catchment area, Mount Holly, Bordentown, and from all over central and southern New Jersey, with every variety of illness from trivial to fatal, young and old, male and female. Sometimes there were two of us on duty, but I was solo the night we got a call around midnight from a desperate mother in Lakehurst, New Jersey, the Naval Air Station that had been the scene of the Hindenburg disaster.

Her child, a 3-year-old, had the croup and was having trouble breathing. We told her to come quickly. The child's condition worsened on the way, and on arrival she was practically unable to breathe, her glottis essentially blocked by inflammation and edema, tiny chest heaving desperately and ineffectually. I was a bit desperate myself, because what the child had to have immediately was either emergency intubation or a tracheotomy. I had never done either, having only witnessed and assisted at a few, and the ER was not set up for such surgery.

I picked her up and ran with her up the long corridor to the surgery suite, hoping to find someone there to do the procedure or help me to do it. Providentially, I encountered Colonel Buesing, Chief of Surgery, and Captain Waggoner, Chief of Anesthesiology, coming through the doors of the operating room just the moment I arrived, the fearful mother panting a few yards behind. The surgeons had just finished an emergency appendectomy. I practically threw the little girl into their arms and followed them into the surgery, where they did a quick and uneventful tracheotomy, saving a life.

I stumbled back into the small waiting area I had blindly run through a few minutes before. There was the young mother, pale with dread. I paused briefly and told her, "Ma'am, your child is going to be fine." Then I returned to my duties in the ER.

Well, she thought I had saved her daughter. She wrote a wonderful letter to her congressman, who passed it up the line until it reached the Surgeon General, who sent it onto President Eisenhower, who signed an individual presidential citation crediting me with a heroic act. I learned this a couple of months later at the quarterly meeting of the entire hospital staff, having simply been told beforehand that it was important for me to attend. There, several hundred persons of all rank, including the Commanding General of Fort Dix, Gen. Bergquist and his gentle wife, both of whom I knew and liked from having made house calls to their splendid quarters. The hospital CO read out the citation, followed by applause from the audience.

Mortified, I made my way to the podium, took the microphone and told what actually happened. Everyone smiled indulgently, and afterward, Gen. Bergquist put his arm around my shoulders and said, "Atta boy, Al – spread it around."

Another ER episode was merely painful. A black career sergeant brought in his two or three-year-old son with hands that had been scalded in hot water. He reported that the child had pulled the hot water off the stove or some such explanation for what was an obvious case of child abuse. In due course, there was a trial in a New Jersey civil court. I was called as a witness. The sergeant tried to take the blame for it, but under examination the prosecution was able to prove that the wife, the baby's mother, had done it. The sergeant wasn't even around when it could have happened. The wife was a good-looking, very well groomed, haughty black woman, narcissistic and contemptuous of us all. She got two years in prison. I've always marveled at the sergeant and his motivation. He was a good, solid career man, but willing to sacrifice his career and go to jail for that woman.

Life at Fort Dix was novel and exciting. We were distant from our parents, Diane for the first time; and I had gotten out of Dallas just in time. My mother had moved in across the courtyard from us in the same apartment complex. She relapsed into depression and alcohol abuse not long after we left. It would have been a terrible strain on us and on our young marriage, which was gaining strength from the shared joy of caring for a wonderful baby boy following the recent trauma of firstborn Brenda. While we were away in the Army, Mother's immediately older sister and surrogate mother Aunt Floy managed the situation and got her off to the state hospital in Austin for a long, long stay.

After our initial stay at the Bachelor Officers Quarters, we moved into a Wherry Housing apartment on the base near the hospital. It was a two-story unit similar to our just-vacated Dallas home, though a bit smaller. It lacked air conditioning, an attic fan, dishwasher and washer-dryer. About 50 yards from our backyard, across an asphalt parking lot, was a large, red brick building with washing machines for the apartment dwellers. There were no dryers, just clotheslines behind the apartments where the laundry froze during cold weather. Diane and I discussed which would come first, a washer-dryer or a hi-fi set. The matter was readily settled when I had to do the work myself because Diane came down with the flu for a few days.

Once the appliances were paid for, I bought a kit, a Knight amplifier/preamplifier with 10 watts per channel, and built it in the electronics shop under the tutelage of a master electrician. This man, about 60, the Chief of the Maintenance Services, was a second-generation Pennsylvania German who had been apprenticed to the organ-builder trade when he was a child. This required him to learn all about sound systems. He was proud of having built or repaired almost all the older organs in Eastern Pennsylvania. He seemed to know everything about music and electronics, and he grew fond of me and was very patient, helping me understand the diagrams, and teaching me to solder. I went to his shop after supper, working past 10 on many nights. Those were happy hours. The finished set had two speakers, a turntable and modest radio, and it worked well for many years.

We formed close friendships with three couples. Nancy and David Glassner from Milwaukee had two young children. They lived off post, some miles north of Fort Dix in the small town of Bordentown. Dave and Nancy spent an unintended weekend with us the second winter, due to a huge snowfall that came while we were attending a dance at the Officers' Club. We were able to drive our car the few hundred yards to our apartment, partially burying it in a snowbank a short trudge from our door.

Nothing moved in or out of the base for two days and power was lost. We scrambled eggs, heated water on a Sterno stove and made do with candles. The vast area was silent, buried beneath two or three feet of heavy snow with drifts up to six feet and higher. The daily drone of air transports and 7 a.m. blast of F-92s taking off from McGuire and thundering a few hundred feet over our apartment were absent. All quiet.

We got along just fine. Dave and Nancy were able to call home to the kids and babysitter. After two nights, they left and I was able to get back to work.

The local Army newspaper had just featured a story about the airman who had won the prize, a three-day pass, for the best plan for keeping the McGuire Air Force Base runways open in case of a winter storm. When the storm came, the bulldozers were on one side of the airfield and the snowplow blades were on the other side; nothing flew or landed for about 60 hours.

ALBERT D. ROBERTS, MD

The other two couples were Dick and Nelda Romig from California with their two small children, and Stan and Zelda Rosenthal from Miami with one or two small children. The Romigs lived a few doors away in the same complex. We babysat for each other. This did not always go well. Once when we kept little Kim, she fell on her head, but thankfully, there was no permanent damage. Worse for everyone concerned was the time we left Truett with the Romigs so that we could spend two or three days at the Atlantic City "Shore Meetings" of the Society for Clinical Investigation, the American Federation for Clinical Research and the Association of American Physicians. These were the most important research meetings in those years. There is nothing like it today. While Diane and I were in Atlantic City, Truett, just past 2 (this was May 1959) fell ill with the measles. He was a miserable little boy and quite sick. His recovery was worse, first severe otitis media, just as I's had at age 7. Much worse was an ischiorectal abscess, a big pus-filled and very painful infection, probably staphylococcal. This had to be drained surgically. One night, his temperature reached 105. I sat up all night with him. I had some Chloromycetin in the medicine cabinet and started him on that. Stan Rosenthal said later that the Chloromycetin may have been critical to staving off a likely sepsis bloodstream invasion that awful night. Truett was far from cured, however. The abscess returned. Weeks later, after our return to Dallas, the abscess was drained again. This time, Dr. Jerry Stirman of the Department of Surgery left the drains in until the abscess finally cleared up.

This episode was the only really bad thing that happened the whole time, although it was a very tough time for Diane, especially the first six months or so. At nadir, her weight dropped from her usual 115 pounds to 103. I don't recall any complaints, let alone tears or recrimination. After we settled into our new way of life, we had some enjoyable times.

New York and Philadelphia were both about 45 minutes away. There was convenient bus service to New York, and Philadelphia was an easy and pleasant drive. During our time at Fort Dix, my Aunt Merle and her second husband, Tom Vic Tirado, lived in New York in a lavish apartment purchased with Aunt Merle's wealth, inherited from her first husband, Dale W. Moore. Dale, a suave and colorful wildcatter, was more than 30 years older than Merle; Tirado was 10 or 12 years younger. Their Park Avenue penthouse was furnished with unrestrained extravagance. I recall Egyptian and classical Greek figures. Tirado had constructed a theater with the finest available sound system, gigantic Klipsch speakers, and projection equipment. For a couple of years they convened a celebrated New York salon that included a number of the glitterati of the day, Leonard Bernstein, the actor Laurence Harvey and his covey. After a couple of years, Merle decided this was not her sort of crowd and moved back to Houston, divorcing Tom. Two more expensive, failed marriages followed, but that did not deter her from supporting the education of many of her nieces and nephews. She was a "river to her people" to the last.

While Merle was living in New York, it was a bonanza for Diane, baby Truett and me. We had a cozy guest bedroom to ourselves, and their live-in houseboy, cook and factotum, an elderly Chinese man, babysat Truett, for whom he seemed to have real affection.

It was a golden age in New York. The international style of architecture was fresh, new, and dazzling: The Seagram's Building, Mies van der Rohe's great legacy, and the Lever Brothers skyscraper. The city was clean, safe and not expensive. We had a beloved neighborhood French restaurant, the Paris-Brest, 50th and Ninth, by the docks. A tiny place, seating maybe two dozen plus some singles at the small but classic zinc bar. French sailors and knowledgeable New Yorkers frequented it. A fellow Army doctor who was a psychiatrist and Manhattan native put me onto. At the Paris-Brest, we first beheld a Frenchman, wearing a beret and eating asparagus with his fingers. There I first ate escargot and frog's legs, and learned what a proper onion soup was like and even a little bit about wines. Madame, the proprietress, was an ancient French lady indifferent to her age and advanced osteoporosis. The kitchen, the size of a walk-in closet, was filled with a large black iron stove and two very busy and agile cooks. These three comprised the staff.

Nelson Rockefeller was governor. John Lindsey was mayor. On radio, we had the great monologist Jean Shepherd, and on TV, David Susskind and his innovative "Open End," so named because the discussions went on until they were over, even if they stretched on well after midnight. We were watching the memorable night that he hosted Dorothy Parker, Norman Mailer and Truman Capote. Parker was near the end of her career, Capote in mid-stride, and the youthful Mailer seemed a bit abashed in their presence, being newly famous for The

Naked and The Dead. They talked about writing and writers. The Beats came up, with Mailer mentioning Kerouac. That's when Capote lisped, tiny fingers typing air, "Oh, I've read Kerouac. He has a certain pace, a certain sheen, but so much of it is just ... TYPING."

There was also the classical music station, WQXR, revelatory to me. And of course, we went to the great museums in New York and Philadelphia. Diane's parents came up in '57 and '58. Fred Truett was president of the National Wholesale Drug Association and presided, at their national meeting in March of 1958, just at Truett's first birthday. The Truetts paid for (more likely it was the NWDA) a room adjacent to their suite in the Waldorf Towers, the only time I had been there since 1939. Baby Truett was a huge hit in his red corduroy jumper, just walking.

Several of Fred's associates were attentive to Diane and me during our stay at Fort Dix. The Strausses had us out to their summer place in Asbury Park on the Jersey Shore, a large handsome Victorian house with a fine, green lawn. Mr. Strauss grilled steaks outdoors, not the only time I have suffered to see prime sirloin ruined with smoke. But they were splendid hosts. Also wonderfully generous to us were Ivan and Mary Elizabeth Combs. We stayed a weekend with them in Scarsdale. I played tennis with Ivan at the Westchester Country Club, not well, but appreciatively. The high point of that visit was the drive through narrow rural lanes at the peak of a glorious fall to the Fox Hill Inn in Connecticut for a wonderful dinner. The beauty of the New England forest and the quiet elegance of the inn more than compensated us for the way Ivan had hurled his Buick through wood and dale.

We made motor trips to Washington, D.C., where we visited Jere Mitchell doing his tour at the National Institutes of Health (NIH) and also Floyd and Margie Rector at the NIH. Then we journeyed to visit Dick and Ginny Portwood at Duke Medical School. After that, it was across the Smokies to stay with my father and Lora on Signal Mountain, above Chattanooga.

There were regular motor trips to Princeton, to New Hope and Bucks County, as well as Philadelphia; and to little villages around and about New Jersey, as well. I shopped at J. Press in Princeton and became a convinced Ivy League convert. There was a classical music shop nearby where we bought our first classical records to play on my new stereo. I was most pleased while shopping for records at the music

A LIFETIME IN MEDICINE

store when a clever salesman, encouraging me to buy, reminded me that they offered a discount for faculty members.

Lasting Images

Certain images remain strong in memory: The old career sergeants nearing retirement, many quietly alcoholic. Once in the early mornings in the ER, the sergeant on duty and I were alone. He was desultorily pushing a floor mop around, and I was intoning about the sometimes poor physical condition of inductees from the big northeastern cities, some of whom had never walked more than a few blocks nor had any form of physical exercise. The old sergeant with the mop listened to me awhile then said, "I don't know, Doc, some of those boys did pretty well in Korea."

At the other end of the spectrum were the splendidos, the officers. We had a visit from a close childhood friend, Lynn Harding, then an Air Force Major stationed at Wright Field in Dayton, Ohio, and charged with the top-secret assignment of monitoring Soviet missile programs. He touched down at McGuire AFB on his way to a regular briefing of the Senate Intelligence Committee and Pentagon senior officers. Lynn loved the Air Force, and he was all military rectitude and attitude. A chain smoker, he had a massive heart attack a few years later and was invalided out of the Air Force. Although devastated for a time, he made a second and equally successful career for himself as a high school math instructor in Austin, Texas. His damaged heart beat on until it terminally failed about 30 years after the original episode.

Lynn was what a career officer should be. And the most dazzling example I ever beheld up close was Gen. Heintges, three stars as I recall. On a normal weekday morning, like any other morning, I began my day by entering my small office on the Critically Ill Ward. There, standing 6 feet 2 inches, was General Heintges in sharply starched and pressed infantry field kit, the sky blue silk infantry scarf at his neck exactly matching his eyes. He had close-cropped gray hair and a lot of white teeth. At his side was an aide-de-camp, a captain somebody.

I was very surprised, having had no advance notice and not enough coffee. I think I mumbled something like, "Oh! Hi, uh, sir?" The general just chuckled. I can't remember what they were there for, some simple question or a request having been directed to me, probably by Gen. Bergquist. Gen. Heintges was on his way to take command in South Vietnam. The buildup was beginning.

At the end of June 1959, I received my honorable discharge. We three loaded up the '57 Ford Ranch Wagon and took one long last drive through the Smokies to Chattanooga for a visit with Pop and Lora, and then home to Dallas. Diane was by then in her third trimester. She had been nauseated the previous December, driving through the Smokies, her pregnancy confirmed soon after.

So a decisive interval in the story of our lives ended. We had lived in a very different part of the country, completely independent of what had gone before, save for doctoring and parenting. The utterly new environment had caused even mundane activities to seem new and fresh. We had new challenges and an array of exciting cultural opportunities and new friends. It was difficult at first for Diane, but she showed the sturdy stuff that Twitchells and Truetts were made of. It was easier for me. I was a doctor doing what I knew how to do in the company and ready-made fellowship of doctors everywhere and in circumstances much pleasanter than the stress of a Parkland house officer's life. We both grew in maturity, confidence and independence. Diane had a little crush on Nelson Rockefeller. We had left Dallas two years before, conventional middle-class Texas conservatives. We returned with a much more critical awareness and a more liberal orientation.

Shortly after we returned to Dallas, I received a Commendation Ribbon and Medal in the mail with a letter from Lieutenant Colonel Blohm explaining that it had arrived too late for the formal presentation. The medal stands today in its Lucite case in my study. It is not one of the great medals, but you can't do a lot better without coming under fire, and I'm quietly proud of it. I wear the little green, gold and white lapel pen on July 4th and November 11th, whenever I can remember to do so.

Chapter 5

Saving Lives and Killing Dogs

The next chapter in my professional life was brief and inglorious, in contrast to previous years. Starting July 1, 1959, I was once again a research fellow and low in the pecking order. I could have gone directly into private practice or gone anywhere for additional specialty training. If I had been single, I might have chosen a career in the Army, but Diane and I both wanted to return to Dallas, and I still had some notion of attempting a career in academic medicine.

I had been a National Institutes of Health Fellow in Diseases of Metabolism, 1956-57, but had done no research, being preoccupied as Chief Resident. At the Atlantic City meetings in May of 1958, Dr. Seldin asked me what my future plans were. I replied that I would like to do another year of Fellowship. Dr. Seldin hesitated momentarily, then said he would "take another chance" on me.

Soon after arrival back in Dallas, I went to see Dr. Seldin, who arose amid the familiar, immense clutter and deceptive disorder of his office and cordially welcomed me. He told me I was to take my time settling back in, do some reading, talk to other members of the Department, and think about what I wanted to do. He, of course, already knew what he had in mind for me.

I was given two assignments: To help develop a hemodialysis program, and, in association with this, a research project focusing on the effect of hemodialysis on certain aspects of kidney function. The research project rather quickly collapsed owing to logistical complexities and flaws in the experimental design. In contrast, the patient care aspect of the project, the hemodialysis service, went well.

Though it was demanding, lives were saved, and a regular hemodialysis service was established for the first time at Parkland Hospital.

The Travenol Twin Coil artificial kidney arrived in July of 1959, simultaneously with my return from the Army. It was the DC3 of hemodialysis due to its relative simplicity, reliability and suitability for mass production at a reasonable cost. The apparatus looked like your grandmother's washing machine, which it was, in a sense, with its major components having been adapted from production washing machines. Its operation was relatively simple compared with other dialysis contraptions because the twin coils, which contained the dialysis membranes, were disposable. Thus, they did not have to be laboriously assembled and disassembled, as was characteristic of the other, paleotechnic devises of that era, the Kiil Horizontal Plate Dialyzer and the Skeggs-Leonard rotating drum, which looked like a Marcel Duchamps design.

Vascular access was crucial to a hemodialysis treatment. You had to connect to an artery, typically a small artery in the wrist, to get blood out of the patient and through the dialysis machine, and to a vein in order to get the blood back into the patient. This required minor vascular surgery each time a dialysis was performed. Surgeons were seldom available, so we did the operations ourselves, not in the operating room with bright lights, swift nurses and sumptuous arrays of sparkling steel, but there in the cramped, hot dialysis room on 6 South. I did most of the work myself and became rather proficient at vascular access.

A treatment took six hours, plus an hour each to hook up and close up, and the physician had to be in virtually continuous attendance. We did only acute dialysis; chronic life-supporting dialysis was many years in the future. We treated acute renal failure, poisonings and acute electrolyte (blood chemistry) disturbances such as the man who came into the ER about 2 a.m. totally paralyzed, except for shallow respirations from acute hyperkalemia, serum potassium, 10 mg. per liter, twice the normal level. This near-fatal episode was likely caused by acute rhabdomyolysis, damaged muscle tissue releasing potassium into the blood. Although the cause was never established, we suspected that it was due to pressure from prolonged immobility coupled with acute alcohol intoxication.

Much less demanding was peritoneal dialysis, which like hemodialysis, was in a primitive stage of development. Today's smartly

A LIFETIME IN MEDICINE

packaged ready-to-go kits were several decades away. We did both kinds of procedures regularly. The renal consult service was also a source of satisfaction. These activities and the acquisition of the skills required to perform them were for me some of the best things about that year.

My second responsibility was to do research. After my original project, the effect of hemodialysis on kidney function, proved impractical, I was assigned to work with my classmate Floyd Rector on the bicarbonate experiment. Floyd had had two years at the National Institutes of Health in Bethesda, working under Dr. Robert Berliner, a world leader in renal physiology, and was already an Assistant Professor and well-embarked on a brilliant academic career.

Salient among its many vital functions, the kidney maintains the level of acidity in body fluids. This is does by several mechanisms, but the most important mechanism of controlling acidity on a moment-to-moment basis involves the balance of carbon dioxide, maintained by respiration and by sodium bicarbonate levels, which are controlled by the kidney. The exact relationship between the level of carbon dioxide (CO_2) and kidney bicarbonate reabsorption was unclear. That relationship was what our experiment was about. The studies were performed on dogs.

The dogs were obtained from the pound and kept in cages in the animal center until their day came. Early in the morning on the day of an experiment, one would be brought into the lab, placed on the operating table and quickly anesthetized. We would then intubate and catheterize the dog and insert arterial and venous bloodlines.

The CO_2 level in the animal's inspired air would be progressively increased as we measured the response in blood and urine at regular intervals. We found that the kidney's response to rising levels of blood CO_2 and the resulting rise in acidity levels was to increase instantaneously the rate of bicarbonate reabsorption. We measured the kidney's response to a wide range of CO_2 levels.

Our research yielded a very nice paper that was published in the Journal of Clinical Investigation and was widely cited for years, most notably in Robert F. Pitt's textbook Renal Physiology.

As for the dogs, the levels of acidity were so damaging to their systems that they were euthanized at the end of the experiment.

Because we were illuminating basic physiologic processes of value to mankind, we did not worry too much about the dogs' fate. We made sure that the dogs were handled humanely, and we knew that had they remained at the pound they would be euthanized there. Nevertheless, even after more than a half century, I'm still a little uneasy, remembering the dogs.

Spring came. I knew that I was not going to fit in. I went to Dr. Seldin and told him that I had decided to go into private practice. His response was unambiguous and eager, "I'll help you!" I put aside my wistful dreams of a life in the Groves of Academe, took stock of my skills in both internal medicine and nephrology, a nascent subspecialty in great demand, and concluded that private practice was the more appropriate path for me at that time.

A Decade Remembered

And so the first decade of my life in medicine rounded to a close, and a new and challenging horizon appeared. I had been a medical student, intern, resident and fellow all at Southwestern and Parkland, plus the two stimulating years as an Army doctor. I had been a good medical student but top tier only in the third year when I had A's in Medicine and OB/GYN and B's in the other courses. It was enough to qualify me for the Medical Honorary Society, Alpha Omega Alpha.

As a house officer, I had endured the crucible learning experience of Parkland, borne the responsibilities, matured rapidly and probed my limits.

I have described the vivid personalities of great teachers who taught me and my classmates to be doctors.

Yes, good men (and woman, Gladys Fashena) all, and reverently remembered. But that decade and the three that follow really belong to Don Seldin.

This memoir is about me and not about Don, but he towers over the era from 1951 onward like a colossus. It was like being a baritone in the Sinatra era. It didn't matter whether you liked him or not; either way you had to decide to sing like him or sing some other way. Still a vivid presence in his late 90s, he is rightly regarded as the father of UT Southwestern.

A LIFETIME IN MEDICINE

He found a feeble school in World War II plywood shacks when he arrived in 1951. He nearly went back to Yale. A few of Dallas' leading physicians persuaded him to stay, all credit to them. Throwing himself into the task, he scolded, badgered, charmed and threatened – whatever it took – to build, over the ensuing decades, one of the greatest Medical Departments in the world. And then, mirabile dictu, he voluntarily stepped down in 1985, to the surprise of all. Most of us thought he so deeply identified with his job and the Department that it would be impossible for him to surrender it to another while yet he breathed. Perhaps not the most original thinker of his era, he was a superb and exhausting critic. He was an excellent clinician and superb teacher. His rigorous intellect, powerful presence, singular verbal style and awesome energy permeated and transformed UT Southwestern.

When young he could be cruel, often saving his worst verbal abuse for his favorites. Crueler still was it to be ignored. So there were casualties, and all who were with him on the long march nurse some scars and perhaps some lingering ambivalence. But always there was this saving back-story: that we were all engaged in a noble enterprise, that nothing less than our best effort would do. He was and is genuinely warm and affectionate.

Always there was poetry, Yeats, Shakespeare, Blake. In the early years, he liked to quote the great lines from "On Milton" by Blake:

> "I will not cease from mental fight,
> Nor shall my sword sleep in my hand
> Till we have built Jerusalem
> In England's green and pleasant Land."

Now, Texas is not England, Dallas is not Jerusalem, and God knows Seldin is not Milton, but that was how he felt. That was how we all felt. And here is the last of the poetry, at least for now. That first decade, the 1950s, is nicely rendered in this little parody, to be sung to the tune of an old Christian children's hymn, two verses that came to Charlie Baxter*, stumbling about the corridors of the old Parkland past midnight:

ALBERT D. ROBERTS, MD

Donald loves us, this we know
Dr. Seldin told us so.
We are weak and he is strong.
He is right and we are wrong.
Yes, Donald loves us,
Yes, Donald loves us,
Yes, Donald loves us,
Because he told us so.

*Charles R. Baxter had almost two years of internal medicine training before being drafted. On return, he began a residency in surgery, eventually becoming a world leader in the care of burns. Charlie died in 2005, full of honors – and nicotine.

Chapter 6

1960 to 1975
Adventures in Exile

Like Alcibiades in Persia, my 15 years in exile were not at all bad, although they were rough at the beginning and at times along the way. In 1960, success in private practice was far from assured; competence alone was no guarantee. Before the coming of Medicare in 1966 and the evolution of widespread health insurance, good internists, some who had been my teachers, took five or seven years to become fully established. It was usual to borrow from the bank if you lacked private resources, as I did.

Most people stayed away from doctors as much as they could. Preventative medicine, except for vaccinations and the Pap test, was rare, and periodic health examinations were a luxury item reserved for the wealthy. In those days, fees were subject to the operation of a free-market system, which meant that you could determine your own fees and charge what the market would bear, if you chose. The leading internists in that distant time had incomes equivalent to the seven-figure emoluments of today's princes of procedures -- ophthalmologists, gastroenterologists, interventional radiologists, cosmetic surgeons, interventional cardiologists, electrophysiologists and the like.

On the other hand, if you joined a busy doctor or group, you could be established sooner and feel more secure. Then there was the matter of hospital privileges. The most competitive, and hence most desirable, hospitals had closed or restricted medical staffs. There were two avenues to admission to the Baylor Hospital staff: either you joined an established staff member or group, or you provided a service or a function that the hospital needed and lacked. Eager to succeed and financially insecure, I seized upon both routes: I joined two busy internists, and I started the Baylor artificial kidney service.

My new friend, Dr. Bryan Williams, himself a recent entry into the Baylor private practice constellation, suggested that I talk to Drs. Herndon and Galt, who had a thriving practice with offices downtown in the Medical Arts Building. I already knew Dr. Herndon, who had been one of my town attending physicians during my residency, and I knew who Dr. Galt was.

We met, got along well, and, after a few weeks of negotiation and some hesitation on my part, came to an agreement.

I'd had some inchoate trepidations, nonspecific and subjective, and since I could not say what they were, I brushed them aside.

I have often thought about the alternative, borrowing the money to start a solo practice and then building my own group. As things turned out, I could readily have done that, but I didn't know it. Besides, to be honest, I hadn't the foggiest notion how to manage a practice. This is still true of medical education. Only Family Practice actually teaches its trainees how to run an office and manage a practice.

We struck a deal: I would provide my own office furnishings and would be provided with a fully equipped examining room. My salary of $600 a month would be repaid when my net income surpassed that amount. The $600 was on the low side even at that time, but I had a fear of debt, and furthermore, was not sure whether things would work out. If they didn't, I wanted to be able to walk away. In a few months, my monthly salary increased to $800, which more approximated our needs. At the end of the first year, I had grossed about $16,000. Overhead in those days was much lower, well under 40% of earnings.

Re-entry Shock

The Dallas to which we returned in July 1959 was not the Dallas we had left two years before. Diane and I were astonished at the change in the political climate. When we left in 1957, almost everyone was sort of conservative, including us, but not rigid or doctrinal. We returned, having taken a turn to the left, to find that half our acquaintances had joined the John Birch Society and the rest were tainted. At the first dinner party we went to, I was shocked to find myself defending (one) public schools (two) the public health services

A LIFETIME IN MEDICINE

and (three) social security – in short, everything that holds society together.

The itinerate Australian fear merchant Fred Schwartz came to town, terrifying the faithful with doomsday rhetoric and color slides illustrating the global reach of the international communist conspiracy. The peroration culminated with a prophecy. "They will come after you, the elite, first. Very soon a jack-booted communist thug will kick down your front door, place a snub-nosed .45 against the side of your head and blow your brains out."

There was serious talk of privatizing the Army. Everywhere we went we encountered this sort of rogue rant. Communists infested the federal government, the schools, and all major institutions; the takeover was expected any day. I knew people who were burying guns and ammunition in their backyard, preparing for the inevitable coming battles. When Kennedy was killed and Governor Connelly wounded, we thought, as did many others, that someone we knew had probably done it. Lee Harvey Oswald came as a relief.

Like a universal cathartic, the assassination effectively ended this era of public paranoia in the community that we knew. Everyone got down off their stilts or at least shut up. Many transferred their zeal to religion; others simply subsided into a more rational outlook, and a measure of tolerance returned to public and private discourse.

Politics aside, it was not a bad time at all. We had a wonderful family life. Hillary was born August 20, 1959, a delightful baby, blonde and blue-eyed, nearly always jolly and not as demanding as her brother had been those first few months. She started sleeping through the night the day the postnatal homecare nurse's tour was up.

We rented a small white-framed house on Colgate, a block west of St. Michael's Episcopal Church. It had three small bedrooms, one bathroom, and a nice, fenced backyard. A little more than a year later, after my entry into private practice, we bought our first house. It was slightly larger, brick veneer, also three bedrooms, one bath, on Northwood just west of Preston Road. This house had a carport on the alley and a detached room adjacent, ideal for my study. There was a small patio, giving way a backyard enclosed on two sides by thick, tall hedges. The price was $16,500.

On one side lived Alan and Vee Maxwell, Alan was a literary figure of some importance, editor of the Southwest Review. I did a couple of reviews for him and wish I'd kept on. On the other side lived a large, raffish family named Cook, with four active young ones.

We had a supper club that met monthly. It had begun in the '50s, when we were all newly married and just learning about food and wine. The original four couples were Ed and Norma Acker, George and Gloria Nicoud, Peter and Barbara Wiggins and us. We took turns hosting. I blush to recall some of the experiments we tried on each other. I recall one of my sins: Sazerac cocktails before supper. After one of these stiff New Orleans drinks, it didn't matter much what was served for dinner. After dinner, we played charades. Diane was always the champ, and hilarity reigned.

While Diane and I were away during my two years in the Army, Dick and Rita Bass took our place, so there were five couples on our return. The club became much more sophisticated. Meals and wines improved.

Private Practice Arrangements

Drs. James H. Herndon and Jabez Galt had a suite of offices on the fifth floor of the old Medical Arts Building, which stood on the corner of Pacific and Ervay Streets, adjacent to the Republic Bank Building and across the street from the late, equally lamented Dallas Athletic Club. They rented two adjacent rooms to provide space for me. My consultation room was a triangular ex-storage closet with five doors, being about 12-by-eight feet. One door opened into the second room, which was large and sunlit. It had a multipurpose procedures table, overhead operating light, a few cabinets, and a sink in the corner – an ideal room for a surgeon. I am, of course, an internist; but no matter – the space and light made up for the inappropriateness of it, as well as for the idiosyncratic and exiguous consultation room.

The partnership, Dr. Galt and Herndon's personal relationship, the office staff, the office itself and the patients who comprised their practice, initially appeared unexceptionable to my naïve eyes, but problems soon became apparent.

Dr. Herndon was then about 50; Dr. Galt was 42. Both were World War II veterans. Jim had been stationed in Marfa, Texas, at an Army hospital. Jabez had served in the medical unit made up mainly of doctors from Baylor Hospital that went into North Africa in 1942 and was later under fire for 100 days at the Anzio Beachhead. Both were tall and powerful in appearance and personality. Jabez was 6'6" tall with wavy auburn hair rapidly silvering, ice blue eyes and a Hapsburg chin. Jim, about 6'2", had a square chin, athletic physique, and wavy, fading blond hair. They were both good doctors, intelligent, resourceful, energetic, ethical, and devoted to their patients. Both had done some teaching at Parkland Hospital and Baylor Hospital. Jim was my attending physician on teaching rounds at Parkland, and I knew him to be a solid if pedestrian teacher. He had entered private practice in the mid '30s after an internship at Baylor, and was largely self-taught as an Army internist. He successful passed his Boards after the war, when military experience counted toward Board certification and Boards were notoriously tough. Jabez had completed a residency with additional training in pharmacology and a fellowship at the Lahey Clinic in Boston. He joined Dr. Herndon in 1948, and "Herndon and Galt" was a well-known and respected marquee.

There was, of course, the money issue. As with most partnerships, each doctor's percentage of the gross income was calculated annually based on his contribution the previous year. Although Jabez was the higher producer, somehow every year, their share came out equal. The bookkeeper – admirable woman – was Jim's sister-in-law. Her annual rendering of accounts would plunge ever deeper into the earlier years of the partnership when Jim was ascendant, ultimately contriving to demonstrate parity for yet another year. These tense negotiations were agonizing for me. The atmosphere in our office would be fraught for weeks.

Jim had endured poverty as a youngster growing up in Oak Cliff and was very focused on money. When angry, he would unconsciously rattle the coins in his pocket, a dead giveaway. He was also controlling, though this trait was usually exercised in subtle and indirect ways.

The office personnel were suspect, as I soon became aware. The lead RN was paranoid; one of the assistants was a hysteric. There was no command or management structure; employees could play us off against each other.

A resolution occurred after a few years. I became de facto and then de juris the managing partner because Jim and Jabez could seldom agree on any issue, large or small. I had something of a flair for this. I proposed that we share three core personnel: receptionist, secretary and bookkeeper, and that we each have an executive nurse, selected and paid by each one of us. Complaints and conflicts among personnel would come to me.

I proposed that each of us keep his net income while paying an equal share of the overhead. This made for a much better working environment. We moved to spacious new offices on the 13th floor, even hiring an excellent interior decorator, Audrey Price. Audrey spent hours throwing all kinds of patterns and textiles before us, scrutinizing facial expressions and body language more than verbal responses.

I had a succession of excellent RN's, Connie Greisheimer, Barbara Levitz, Pat Morale, and Martha Francis.

Undercurrents remained. Jim could not change his controlling ways, and he grew more morose. Later, in retrospect, I understood that his physical and mental vigor had begun to decline. He had not many more years to live, dying at age 69 of lung disease and perhaps other problems related to his lifetime of excessive tobacco abuse.

I never really stopped feeling like the baby adopted to save a failing marriage. After 11 years of this, I determined to leave and take new space in an attractive one-story clinic a block from Baylor Hospital. At the last minute, almost impulsively, I asked Jabez if he wished to come with me; and, after thinking about it overnight, he agreed. So it was that a new phase in my medical practice began, overall a much more pleasant one.

I must be fair. Both Jabez and Jim always treated me with great generosity. They were strongly supportive of my career development, helped me to build my practice, and did not complain when one of their patients defected to me. "We are all smoothly functioning interchangeable parts of the same machine," Jabez would say. I learned all about private practice from them, owed them both a great deal and remember both fondly.

In many ways, I missed the '60s, was barely aware of the Beatles, and was no more than moderately bemused by the societal storms until the last wavelets crested in the medical schools in the early to mid '70s.

Those 15 years, 1960–1975, were consumed by work: the practice of clinical nephrology intertwined with general internal medicine and teaching. I made attending rounds, teaching students, Interns, Residents and fellows at Parkland, Baylor, the Veteran's Hospital, and later at Presbyterian, which opened in 1966. I was an unpaid volunteer, a "town man," during those years. The VA provided a small stipend plus a significant added benefit in those years, an excellent staff cafeteria.

I am indebted to the VA for the opportunity to do my first kidney biopsy. This requires a brief bit of explanation. First, the procedure was primitive and risky compared to current practice. Second, I had never done one before. In fact, I had never even watched one. In the '50s and '60s, we had the Vim-Silverman needle, adapted from liver biopsy. The procedure was done with the patient prone in his or her regular hospital bed, local anesthetic, of course, and no CT or sonography to guide the operator. The patient held a deep breath, you jabbed the needle into what you hope is the right place in the patient's back, the sheathed biopsy needle blade snipped through the shaft and bit into something. Out came nothing, or a tiny piece of kidney – or sometimes, fat, liver, duodenum, pancreas – or once, all four – a memorable episode in the career of a young resident named Dr. Gary Eknoyan, whom I was supervising during the procedure. The patient was unharmed. Dr. Eknoyan later became a leader in the field of nephrology.

My point is that the technique was tricky, and serious complications could occur. How was it that I, with a year's intensive training in nephrology and a residency in internal medicine, had no experience at all with this indispensable technique? The only person doing kidney biopsies at Parkland during my training was Dr. Norman Carter, a gifted and respected clinician and researcher, but also a rather strange, isolated and reclusive character. More to the point, Norman was not fond of me, doubtless with cause. Whatever the reason, I was never present when Norman did a biopsy, despite my entreaties.

That was the situation one morning in 1960 when the VA house staff presented a veteran with chronic kidney disease, who needed a biopsy for diagnosis. Three previous attempts by VA faculty had failed. The resident at the patient's bedside announced to the ward team that this time a real expert would do the biopsy. He meant me.

I had not expected my first opportunity to come about just so, but was not unprepared. I had read, thought, pictured and mentally practiced it many times.

In the event, it was a success.

My next one was hardly less challenging. The revered and feared Chief of Urology Dr. Harry Spence asked me to do a biopsy on a patient of his. Before nephrologists began doing needle biopsies, urologists did open biopsies, which meant invasive surgery requiring general anesthesia and a few days in the hospital. I knew that Dr. Spence was testing me. He and his young partner, Terry Allen watched while I did it; again, I succeeded. Dr. Spence's approval and support were essential to my success as a consultant. We remained on cordial terms until his death a few years ago in his late 80s.

Between 1960 and 1975, I performed approximately 100 biopsies. Only one resulted in a complication; it was a woman who bled into her kidney a week or so after the procedure from a pseudo-aneurysm, which a clever interventional radiologist patched with a clot of the patient's own blood.

During those years I also gave frequent lectures to practicing physicians, Grand Rounds at Baylor, visits to county societies; presentations to the now long-defunct Dallas Southern Clinical Society Meetings. These activities brought much satisfaction to me, a frustrated would-be academic. I was the first practicing nephrologist in North Texas in 1960, and for a year, the only one. Charlie Austin was the second, joining the internists Drs. Joe Horn and Billie Oliver in 1961.

The first artificial kidney treatment at Baylor Hospital (now Baylor University Medical Center) was around the 1st of July 1960, when a 60-year-old woman from Sulphur Springs, Texas, arrived in critical condition. Her kidneys had shut down following an operation for colon cancer. Her blood urea nitrogen was over 250, more than 10 times normal. She was dialyzed once. The treatment markedly improved her uremic condition. In a few days, she was able to urinate, and she completely recovered.

I had set up the hemodialysis program with the help of some wonderful RNs and support staff. Pat Loomis, RN, came first, followed soon by Sybil Hunter, RN (now Mrs. Gary Eknoyan) and Barbie Montgomery, RN, now Barbie Montgomery-Dossey. Barbie and Larry Dossey are now well-known writers who live in Santa Fe. She is a specialist on Florence Nightingale and nursing subjects. He is the author of many books, the most recent ones focused on the role of faith and prayer in recovery.

These spirited young nurses made the program work, as did the medical Residents. Dr. Austin arrived on the scene in 1961 and quickly took on a large part of the burden. We did not practice together; we had joined different internal medicine groups. In those years, nephrology, particularly hemodialysis, was a "loss leader." There was no Medicare or Medicaid and little enough insurance to support dialysis treatments. Most patients had exhausted their resources by the time they came to end-stage kidney disease. So it was necessary to balance general internal medicine with nephrology in order to make a living.

These early eight-hour hemodialysis sessions required nearly continuous physician attendance. We also did many peritoneal dialyses, a simpler process, although in the days before intensive care units and neat, prepacked kits, it was considerably less simple and efficient than nowadays.

Although much of the dialysis work was de facto pro bono, being the only practicing nephrologists in a huge area enabled Charlie and me to have busy consultation practices. We saw all matter of complex cases, not just kidney diseases, but also lupus and other autoimmune diseases, blood chemistry catastrophes of all kinds, a lot of endocrine problems including diabetic complications, adrenal failure, malignant hypertension, and on and on.

We both did a great deal of teaching. After a few years, Baylor's Chief of Medicine, Dr. Ralph Tompsett, appointed Charlie Director of the Hemodialysis Service and me Director of the Nephrology Lecture Course, weekly teaching sessions that were part didactic and part case presentations and discussion.

I saw all kinds of patients from all over the state and contiguous states. I did peritoneal dialyses on children weighing less than 80 pounds. I still have a battered, old doctor bag given me by the parents of one such child who came from far West Texas for treatments.

It is important to remember, and it is not easy to write about it, that we were not actually sustaining life in those patients whose kidney function had irreversibly failed. We could only provide temporary relief from the terrible manifestations of uremia. There were no techniques for life-sustaining hemodialysis or peritoneal dialysis until the 1970s. After a few hemodialysis treatments, the vascular access sites would be used up. With peritoneal dialysis, complications developed, and I had no patients who requested ongoing repeat treatments beyond a few. So the patients would sicken and die. In many instances, we prolonged the dying.

But we did what we could with what we had, and we saved the lives of many patients with acute or reversible disorders.

There were plenty of challenges and excitement, even humor, such as the day the dialysis team had untimely visitors. We were in the midst of a dialysis treatment, there in our hot, windowless little room in the old Veal Building, the nurse and I, the medical resident and a small covey of student nurses. By and by, I remarked, "A cold beer would sure be good about now." And sure enough, a small, quiet student nurse slipped out of the room, unobserved, and returned in about 20 minutes with a six-pack of Coors. Horrified (this was a really Baptist hospital, where alcoholic beverages were strictly forbidden), I said, "Good Lord! Get that out of sight!"

The words were hardly out of my mouth when the door opened and there stood the hospital's longtime CEO, Boone Powell, Sr. with five or six powerful and influential members of his Board of Directors. They had come to see the marvelous new machine. I can't imagine what sort of tableau vivant we presented there, frozen by surprise, relief and amusement. But the beer was hidden away, and the moment passed. I never asked what happened to the beer.

Perhaps the most painful era in early nephrology came after the development of life-sustaining dialysis techniques by Belding Scribner and his colleagues in Seattle in the late '60s and before the coming of the End Stage Renal Disease Program in the '70s. Scribner had done what now seems a very simple innovation: instead of removing the plastic tubes from the artery and the vein at the end of the treatment, he made a more or less permanent shunt by hooking the arterial and venous tubes together, leaving them in place. It took a few years to work this out to the point where it could be deployed as a routine procedure. The main problems were developing inert materials that could remain attached indefinitely without causing tissue reaction and also controlling infection and clotting. Once these techniques were refined, patients whose kidneys had failed could live for years, often many years, especially if they could survive long enough to receive a transplant.

The cruel dilemma was this: the new technique offered the means to sustain the lives of tens of thousands of people, but most of them could not afford it. The cost, around $25,000 a year when that was twice the median annual income in the nation, was beyond many people's resources; nor could hospitals or physicians provide charity support on the scale posed by this challenge. In addition, patients needed adequate intelligence and a social or family support system.

Around the country, committees of theologians, doctors, laymen, administrators, met to decide who would be treated and who rejected. At Baylor, as I recall, we handled these cases informally; that is, Charlie Austin and I found ways to sustain as many as we could. The others – too old, too sick, too mentally impaired, and too lacking in resources – we treated conservatively, providing what we now call comfort care: diet and drugs to relieve symptoms.

There were some gratifying successes. One is the story of the first patient in Dallas to undergo self-administered home dialysis.

This was in the '60s. Lillian Klemme was about 50 when she abruptly lost all kidney function due to the hemolytic uremic syndrome. There were none of the dialysis centers that we now take for granted, and long-term, life-sustaining programs were not available in hospitals, either. In fact, there was only one place in the world where a patient could go to learn home dialysis: Seattle, home of Dr. Belding Scribner, inventor of the Scribner shunt.

The process was not simple. First, the patient, the patient's family and the doctor were interviewed. One of Dr. Scribner's young associates, Dr. Christopher Blagg, flew to Dallas to check us out. Fortunately, Lillian and Bill Klemme were ideal candidates: stable, intelligent and financially secure. Best of all, Bill was a big, strong, smart engineer. So we were accepted for the hemodialysis training program. There were three days of training in Seattle. The apparatus, the "kidney," was the Kiil horizontal plate dialyzer, a recent Swedish invention. The Kiil required patience and skill. For each of the thrice-weekly treatments, it had to be assembled, and then disassembled following the treatment, all the while maintaining a scrupulously sterile technique. That said, the apparatus had important advantages. In operation it was simple: blood flowed one way between the dialyzing membranes, and dialysis fluid (mixed for each session) flowed the other way; no blood pump was required. The Klemmes mastered the technique readily.

I was taken to Dr. Scribner's office where he greeted me cordially and invited me to lunch. He and his wife lived across Portage Bay from the medical school in a modest traditional sandstone cottage. His 40-foot sailing yacht lay moored at their dock below. Mrs. Scribner, a handsome woman in tweeds, gave us lunch in the breakfast nook, Campbell's tomato soup and grilled cheese sandwiches, exactly the meal that Diane first prepared for me on return from our honeymoon. Beneath the table dozed two immense, elderly, flatulent hounds.

ALBERT D. ROBERTS, MD

Mrs. Scribner drove me back around the bay for my afternoon training session. "Scribbie" followed his habitual custom, paddling back to work in his red aluminum canoe, wearing his raincoat and a yellow hat. I watched him from the dialysis room. A light rain or heavy mist was falling in the gray Seattle afternoon. I was reminded of "The Red Wheelbarrow" by poet William Carlos Williams, and thought:

So much depends upon a bright red canoe glistening in the rain.

Dr. Scribner died in June of 2003, not long after receiving the Albert Lasker Award for clinical research. He shared the award with Willem Kolff, who invented the artificial kidney in Holland during the German occupation. A moving citation was written by a colleague at UT Southwestern, Dr. Joe Goldstein, Nobel Laureate and then Chairman of the Lasker Award Committee.

Dr. Scribner's invention, followed in a few years by Medicare funding for all patients with end-stage kidney disease, made life possible for our patients and life bearable for dawn nephrologists like me. The enormous relief that practical life-prolonging dialysis brought to the physicians and nurses who were attempting to mitigate end-stage kidney disease in those arduous times was never adequately recorded, so far as I am aware.

Lillian Klemme lived on for eight years, eventually dying of heart failure. She and Bill shared her last years traveling in an Airstream trailer, using a Kiil dialyzer for her treatments. Some years after Lillian's death, Bill came to see me. He had remarried and was a contented man. He died just a few years ago. Seeing his obituary in the Dallas Morning News brought it all back to me. I wrote a letter to the editor describing their story. What good people. What an able man.

The second home dialysis patient was an oil company executive who also had an engineering background. We trained him ourselves at Baylor Hospital using the Travenol Twin-Coil Dialyzer that I have already described. They lived less than a mile from my house, and I made house calls; not many needed because he and his wife were also quite competent. He enjoyed several more years of life.

Dallas' first cadaver transplant (now euphemistically referred to as a "recipient from a non-living donor") had also been a patient of mine, a young man who loved the good things in life in abundance, especially food and drink. This was several years before the Scribner shunt. We did a few palliative peritoneal dialysis treatments. This alternative to hemodialysis involved placing a perforated catheter into the abdominal cavity and circulating a balanced electrolyte and glucose solution for several hours. The patient and his parents wanted something better and were willing to risk the very slim chance of success.

Only a few cadaver transplants had been attempted, none in Dallas. However, kidney transplants between identical twins, while uncommon, were successful. In those cases, the kidneys were fresh, and no immunosuppression was required to prevent rejection by the recipient's immune system. Cadaver transplants were quite a different matter: the kidneys were battered, and the patients required toxic immunosuppressive drugs, which were not very effective in those days. The kidneys usually failed, often early on. I counseled against, feeling that palliative treatment would make the young man's last days or weeks more comfortable. The renowned Chief of Experimental Medicine, the one-man department Dr. Arthur Grollman, encouraged the patient to go ahead. And so Paul Peters, Sr., Chief of Urology at Southwestern, a friend and respected colleague, went ahead as soon as a kidney became available. The patient rejected the transplant almost immediately and died soon thereafter, never leaving the hospital. At least it was not a protracted course.

By the mid-1970s, dialysis centers were blossoming all over the country, stimulated by the End-Stage Renal Disease Program, the first and still the only federally funded mechanism supporting organ-specific treatment nationwide. The academic nephrology programs, theretofore sparsely populated by young, research-oriented doctors, rather suddenly blossomed with trainees aiming for careers in the dialysis business, which promised to be lucrative. A vigorous, competent generation of business-savvy young nephrologists developed treatment centers that sustained life for thousands who would have otherwise died much sooner, and, in the process, rapidly enriched themselves. Profit-oriented, efficient groups created many multimillionaire doctors in a few years.

One of the best such outfits was the one in Dallas, formed in 1975 by young men fresh out of training, mainly from UT Southwestern. My colleague Charles Austin was invited to join. I was not. At that time, we were still the only two practicing nephrologists in North Texas, but I was veering more toward a successful general internal medicine practice, while Charlie devoted more time and effort to dialysis. I had to make a decision – I could ask to join the

Southwestern group, start one of my own, or continue to practice general internal medicine with a consulting practice in nephrology. In the event, in that crucial year, 1975, I stuck with my general internal medicine practice. And Charlie Austin shot himself.

Looking back, we were both exhausted and probably both depressed. In large measure, it was the fatigue. Most weeks, I had already worked 40 hours by Wednesday night. There were also long stretches of continuous hospital responsibility, sometimes 40 days or more without missing a day of rounds. And we saw the sickest patients. When the intensive care units were developed (I was on the Baylor committee that helped to develop them), Charlie and I seemed to live in them. We were the first intensivists long before the term and concept were invented. A sour joke was that you couldn't die at Baylor until you had been seen by the chaplain and either Charlie or Al.

And the challenges grew. In 1966 Presbyterian Hospital opened, six or seven miles north of Baylor, so I was covering three hospitals: Baylor, Presbyterian and Gaston, the small, private, non-teaching hospital across the street from Baylor. After an August night in the early '70s when I had mandatory emergency room call at Presby and admitted four very sick patients on top of all of our regular patients, Jim, Jabez and I withdrew from Presby, with some reluctance.

Jabez became the first clinical oncologist in the area, which added another level of duty and challenge. Previously there were one or two pathologists who saw cancer and leukemia patients, not very satisfactorily. As new drugs to treat cancer became available, there was a need for good internists to master them. Jabez was active in the Cancer Society, and his colleagues urged him to take on this nascent subspecialty. For several years, until well-trained clinical oncologists began to emerge from the new programs, we had a busy cancer practice. Familiarity with the new drugs, Cytoxan, methotrexate, 5 fluorouracil, 6-mercaptopurine, Thiotepa, was also helpful in the treatment of autoimmune diseases.

So I was treating cancer and end-stage kidney disease plus all the usual conditions seen by a busy internist. I recall making rounds for our group one December weekend, offering holiday cheer to 15 or 20 patients who would not see Easter. My own in-hospital population peaked at 28 – that was the most I ever had under my own care at one time, though in many of these cases I was a consultant and not the primarily responsible doctor.

A LIFETIME IN MEDICINE

But what of the consequences of decades of overwork? It is nothing like the chronic fatigue syndrome, that poorly understood complex of physical, mental and emotional derangements. What you feel is not so much physical as existential. Burnout is as close as I can come to it. You feel like King Canute battling the tide. There seems to be no end to it. The successes bring no pleasure (after all, it is only what is expected of you), and the failures get you down more. The load just gets heavier; time passes you by. Suddenly one day you're 45. Your wife and children are strangers.

I can't say what Charlie's state of mind was when he took his life, only that our circumstances were very similar. As for my own state of mind, I realized that the offer of a new and different life in academic medical administration couldn't have come at a better time.

Dr. Charles Sprague, President of the UT Health Science Center, and Fred Bonte, Dean of UT Southwestern Medical School invited me to become the Associate Dean for Clinical Affairs. After a few weeks of negotiations, diminishing hesitancy on my part, and despite my wife's misgivings, I took the leap. I took the first month-long vacation of my career, to Italy with the family for a wonderful medical meeting and tour, and then entered my new office at the northeast corner, 11th floor of the new Academic Administration Tower, named for my friend and patient, Margaret McDermott and her husband Eugene; architecture by my friend and patient, Bud Oglesby, on July 1, 1975.

I had been offered the position once before, in 1971, by Dr. Sprague and Doug Lawrason, the dean at that time, and had turned it down after weeks of painful indecision. To return to the medical school as a dean with prospects of advancement, if successful, was powerfully tempting. In the first 11 years of private practice, I had achieved or surpassed my own expectations and was not discontent at that time; still, part of me yearned for academia. The years in private practice always felt like exile, however successful. I thought of Alcibiades, in exile twice, first among the Spartans after the Syracuse disaster and later in Persia. He was feted and honored in both places, yet he yearned for the wine of Athens and the company of Socrates. And so did I.

And yet, here was this private practice I had worked so hard to build. There were challenging cases referred by respected colleagues, personal friends and community leaders. I had enough teaching opportunities to satisfy any would-be academic. Eventually private practice won that round. After weeks of attempted rational analysis, pro and con lists, debates with Diane and with myself, I felt that the private practice experience had not yet been fully realized. Diane, more objective and less emotionally invested, always thought, both then and later, that academic medicine was not right for me.

A Special Way of Listening

Those weeks of introspection in 1971 precipitated my decision to enter into psychotherapy. My perception was that the real reason I did not decide to go to the Medical School was that I was unable to make a decision, consequently staying in harness by default. Part of this disturbing state of mind was the feeling that deep down I didn't really know myself; beneath this "presenting complaint", this conscious or surface symptomatology, I was vaguely aware, lay something much deeper and more complex. It was also becoming apparent to me that my professional success, bought by such arduous travails, was not being rewarded by a commensurate degree of satisfaction or happiness. There were spasms of exaltation wrought by some achievement here, some recognition there and, in my intellectual life, by the intense pleasure of a sudden insight or by having seen an answer or solved a problem that had perplexed others. But mostly, day in and day out, week after week, month after month I just slogged along, despondent, piling task on task, the gulf between effort and satisfaction ever widening.

Furthermore, I wasn't doing a particularly good job as husband and father. We had a stable, happy home, and the children were doing just fine, but that was mainly Diane's doing.

Surrounded by good reasons to be happy, I wasn't. The prevailing mood was one of despondency – seldom really miserable, never actually suicidal, though aware that the path ahead could lead that way.

This was the state of things when I took myself to see Dr. Bill DeLoach, the Acting Chairman of Psychiatry at the Medical School. Bill was a good friend and tennis partner. We referred patients to one another. Himself an eclectic practitioner, he had been in psychoanalysis and was analytically oriented in his approach. After two sessions, he recommended psychoanalysis. This was not a surprise. Once, years before when I was an anxious and depressed house officer, I had consulted Dr. Al Shapiro, who had himself been in analysis, and Al had suggested the same. But on Diane's teacher salary and my resident stipend, that was not realistic at the time.

Clarence Parker, M.D., then in his 50s, had a small suite, a waiting room and consultation room in a discreet little one-story brick professional building on Dickason Street. The magazines strewn about the waiting room were almost all about history. The consultation room might have been 14 by 18 feet, neutral colors, soft light, and comfortable leather couch. A handsome fur throw hung from a coat rack at the foot of the couch. At the window end of the room were Dr. Parker's desk, chair and telephone. At the other end, behind and to the side of the couch, a comfy armchair enfolded Dr. Parker wearing his trademark sandals. No secretary, no electronics. Clarence answered the phone himself and typed his own invoices. His fee was $35 for the 50 minutes. Later it would be raised, but not much.

In this setting, I spent more than 1,100 hours over a five-year period. As Paul Simon famously asks, "Can analysis be worthwhile?" In a general way, it's hard to say because we don't know what we would have been without it. The method is fraught with tautologies and self-fulfilling postulates. Many old Freudian concepts seem ridiculous now, though we can't think about the personality, emotion and neuroses without some recourse to the Freudian topography.

Personally, I wasn't a very good analysand. Deeply distrusting all authority, I wasn't susceptible to transference, and I filled up a year or two of 50-minute hours with small talk and paid attempts to entertain my analyst. Dr. Parker, trained in the Philadelphia School, would "show me no mercy," as he said toward the end of the analysis. By this, he meant that he would not give me the answers that I wanted but was too sullen, infantile or unfocused to work toward. He was impeccably correct. Any truths given me without effort, I would have devalued.

And yet, somehow everything matters. You lie there and listen to yourself month after month, a little nudge, perhaps just a throat cleared, now and then from the business end of the couch, and from time to time things fall into place, and you see and feel something with startling clarity for the first time. My test for truth felt like something I had always known.

Another metaphor I used was that the "aha!" moment was like the bolt of a well-oiled rifle snapping into place.

We would sometimes make good use of dreams. There were three right at the start of the analysis. The night before the first visit, I dreamed I could not find the keys to my white 1967 Mercedes Benz 250SE sedan. This was a slam-dunk for Dr. Parker: I didn't really want to come to the sessions and begin analysis.

The second dream was the Thomas Gainsborough portrait of the "Blue Boy." In my boyhood home in Preston Hollow, Dallas, there had been a similar portrait of my youngest brother John, about age three in blue velvet. Dr. Parker said it meant I would disguise myself in analysis. In the third dream, I was in an old prop-driven airliner. We flew over icy arctic waters and landed in Siberia in a barren field that turned out to be muck like a septic tank or the bottom of an outhouse. But then I entered an old, one-story dimly lit building and inside all was warmth, laughter and welcoming gaiety. This dream, Dr. Parker said, was about analysis: a journey, mysterious and threatening, working through what the analysand always fears is liable to be pretty nasty stuff; then, a warm and happy arrival at the end.

These introductory dreams, facile and obvious, Clarence readily explained, perhaps to engage me in the process. Other later dreams, even two recurrent ones, he turned aside or deferred. One such was a dream of a wonderful classic automobile lying abandoned, overgrown and rusting in an unknown field. Sometimes it was a glorious, cream-colored Mark V Jaguar drop head, green leather, and big bucket headlights. Such a car had briefly belonged to a medical school friend. Other times it was my father's ill-fated 1948 Lincoln Continental convertible, which was abandoned to rust in a field by my brother Bobby. Our father, who was living in Austin near Bobby, could no longer keep it up, nor could Bobby. I knew nothing of this until years later. For me, the dream represented an undifferentiated, forlorn yearning.

In the other recurrent dream, I was flying, energetically flapping my arms like wings, over neighborhood rooftops. This dream was extremely real. I was always a little surprised to awaken and find that it had not been true. Decades later, reading Strozier's biography of Heinz Kohut, I discovered that this dream is typical of the narcissistic personality disorder. At the time, Clarence would tell me that it was because my arms were tired from exercise. At such times, I might feel like a 40-pound fish played on a 10-pound line, but I always thought he knew what he was doing. It would have been better for the process if I had argued about it, but in the end, even well before the end, I stopped having the dream altogether.

A LIFETIME IN MEDICINE

Dr. Parker would never use the words narcissism, complex or neurosis; he used plain, everyday language, however parsimoniously. Depression, yes. It became gradually clear that I had been depressed, or not far from it, at least since the age of three, when my mother was first hospitalized for psychotic depression.

So was it after all worth it? Even allowing for cognitive dissonance – arguing with myself over whether 1,100 paid hours could have been a mistake – I would say so. To begin with, it immediately took some of the edge off my discomfort and somewhat mitigated my worst bouts of misery. While there was no final resolution, I emerged with a workable picture of myself and how I got that way. I was, and am, able to stand a bit apart from myself, with a measure of comprehension, tolerance and, often, amusement.

In a real sense, the analysis has never stopped. While certainly not preserved from foolish mistakes in thought and action, now I can usually understand how such things come about. By thinking back to things I learned on the couch, I can explain them to myself and sometimes enjoy a late-blooming, sudden blink of insight.

The other benefits, very real and important to me, involve my family life and more broadly, my life as a social being, and my professional life. In the years before the start of treatment and for the first year or so of treatment, I was often unhappy and making my family unhappy. I was too seldom cheerful, outgoing, supportive, too much centered on myself. My professional work went reasonably well; the practice and the workload grew apace. I even continued to take on extra projects. Along with the nephrology course and Baylor and Parkland teaching rounds, I developed the Baylor University Hospital Advanced Seminars in Internal Medicine, a three-day paid continuing education course for practicing physicians. In other words, I was doing more and enjoying it less and less.

There is little doubt in my mind that both my professional life and marriage would have deteriorated had not I entered therapy. The professional self that emerged from formal therapy has continued to mature along avenues that likely would not have been forthcoming otherwise, and consequently all of my experiences as a physician and in various public roles have been richer, deeper and more rewarding than they otherwise would have been.

The benefits of psychoanalysis have nowhere been more apparent to me than in the consultation room; that is, in my encounters with individual patients. It is a special way of listening deeply and an innate feeling of how to respond. Along with that, I learned an added measure of patience and tolerance and, at its best, the ability to take a wide range of patients just as they are and help them get to the next place – symptom relief, insight, acceptance of reality – and to feel a little more in charge of themselves than when they came in.

Many good doctors learn these things on their own, as they mature, without years on the couch. Maybe I would have done so on my own, but I know I would not have been able to feel so deeply the satisfactions afforded me by these experiences, and certainly I would never have been able to stay in harness into my 80s.

To have found, with Ruskin, that "all men have poetry in their hearts," and to have found this truth at the extremities of people's lives, may be the best thing I have done.

Chapter 7

The Smiling 45-Year-Old Associate Dean

And so it was that when the second offer of the Associate Dean position came in 1975, I knew myself well enough to make the decision with confidence. I considered the good things I would leave behind: well-respected partners and an elegantly comfortable office. Over 15 years, I had built a rewarding private practice and was an active consultant with ample opportunities for teaching.

Yes, I had overworked and wanted to try something entirely new, and another chance like this was not likely to come after age 45. But what an era in medicine it was! Although we little perceived its evanescence at the time, it was the high noon, the apogee, of internal medicine, compared to the times that have followed.

And then there were the patients, by then around 1,500. There were a few I would be glad to be rid of, but many more had become my friends and, to no small extent, my mentors. My personal, emotional, and intellectual investment in many of these relationships was deep and binding. I cared about them. I also really liked Baylor Hospital and had pleasant and efficient working relationships with professional colleagues and a fine house staff.

In the end, the allure of academic medicine won out. I had lain awake many nights. Always there had been this yearning, related, I suspect, to an unconscious wish to reconstitute my nuclear family and to get it right this time. In the end, the decisive question was, "What if I don't do it?" So, having used my head as much as I could, I went with my heart. However, I kept an escape hatch, retaining a small private practice one half day a week in my old office, shared with my generous and tolerant partner, Dr. Jabez Galt.

The McDermott Administration building, the "Tower," commands the northeast corner of McDermott Plaza. My new corner office on the eleventh floor faced north and east. It was amazingly elegant and spacious, a fine big desk and executive chair, a conference table seating eight, and two walls lined with bookshelves. Behind my desk was the Herman Miller wall organizer I had brought with me from my private office. I had an antique couch from Diane's family, circa 1900, that had been refinished and used in my previous offices as additional seating for group meetings and as a most welcome place for a quick nap.

There were at that time just four large corner offices on the eleventh floor. Within this regal perimeter, the support staff labored, and the building core housed elevators, stairs and facilities. The other associate deans were Bryan Williams for Students, Ron Estabrook for the Graduate School, and John Schermerhorn for Allied Health.

I felt somewhat less significant than my surroundings, but it was exciting, stimulating, and very different from clinical practice. I had title, rank, tenure, a splendid office, adequate salary, and excellent colleagues. I reported to Dean Fred Bonte and to President Charles Sprague. They occupied the twelfth floor, along with the large Board Room. We worked well together. Genial and gregarious, Charlie was always the largest presence in any gathering. Fred was forthright, vigorous, humorous, and, at times, impulsive. Somehow, the three of us made for a good mix.

There was a challenging array of clinical issues piled on my desk, "clinical" meaning relationships critical to the faculties, facilities, students and Residents from the third year of medical school through residency.

A glance through the work journal I kept as I was getting a grip on my duties and responsibilities reveals that the most pressing items in my portfolio had to do with relationships with teaching hospitals. First and foremost, I served as the UT Southwestern representative to Parkland, and also to Baylor Hospital, Presbyterian Hospital, St. Paul's and Methodist Hospitals. We had problems with them all, but chiefly with Parkland and Presbyterian.

In fact, my position, Associate Dean for Clinical Affairs, had been created by Dr. Sprague to deal with these matters, or reconfigured for that purpose. During the year before my recruitment, conflicts had escalated to the point of being aired publicly in newspaper articles and critical editorials. Bad press for everyone. An assembly of leaders from the various institutions met to resolve conflicts and coordinate plans and goals. I functioned as liaison and executive secretary, arranging meetings and agendas. The group met for a few years until the issues subsided, along with the overt rancor. From my perspective, we met until everybody got bored with the issues, or the issues just became obsolete or went underground. The assembly's functions were more or less folded into the North Texas Council of Hospitals.

There continued to be serious conflicts between UT Southwestern and Parkland, the county's charity hospital. The natural tension occurred because the two institutions, while yoked together by the mission of patient care, served separate masters. A Board of Managers appointed by the County Commissioners governs Parkland and the Dallas County Hospital District, and their goal is to provide care for the indigent at the lowest possible cost. The University of Texas Board of Regents governs the Medical School, and it has a threefold warrant: caring for patients, training physicians and conducting scientific research.

Over the decades, the tension has produced mainly creative and positive results. The late '70s and early '80s were a bad time, however. The hospital was struggling with decaying facilities, inefficient administration and suspect accounting.

Rescue came in the form of Ralph Rogers.

Ralph was a formidable leader with a reputation for saving failing or threatened entities. He was a key figure in salvaging the Dallas Symphony and the Public Broadcasting System when they were threatened with extinction during the Nixon Administration. When he took over as President of the Parkland Board of Managers, the first thing he did was to sequester himself for about six weeks with all the administrative records that he could command. When he emerged, he knew more about Parkland than anyone before or since. I witnessed firsthand the basis of his success: an unparalleled command of information and a dominating personality wrapped in a brilliant mind. I never saw him in any group that he did not control, large or small. He also controlled events. Parkland's President and CEO at that time was Jack Price, who had made a good start years before, but whose energies in recent years had been largely consumed by playing the county commissioners and the school administration off against one another, thus maintaining himself in office while allowing the hospital to decay. If the commissioners got on him, he would say to us, "Look what those S.O.B.s are trying to do to us!" Conversely, if we applied pressure, he would entreat the commissioners to intervene.

But County Judge Gary Weber appointed Ralph Rogers to be Parkland Board Chairman, and such was Ralph's prestige and community support that together they were able to reform and rescue the hospital.

Ralph saw early on that Mr. Price would have to go, and he took pains to lay the groundwork. That was where I came in. One day Ralph invited me to lunch at his Trinity Industry's executive dining room. I knew this lunch meant some sort of challenge for me.

Ralph and his wife Mary Nell fetched me in a capacious navy blue Cadillac. Mary Nell was chauffeuring, and I reposed in the back with Ralph on the deeply quilted black leather seat.

"Which way do you want to go, dear?" Mary Nell asked.

"Anyway you like, dear," he replied.

"All right, I'll go up to Record Crossing and take a left and ..."

"Oh no," came the prompt rejoinder, "That's not the way to go. Let me tell you the right way."

I received my mission over a tasty lunch of beef burgundy, prepared by Ralph's private chef, Jean-Claude Prevot.

The fact that I worked for the School and not for Ralph mattered not in the least. Ralph expected me to prepare a list of particulars to fortify his position in case Jack Price declined to bail out with the generous parachute Ralph had prepared for him. As it worked out, Price took the deal and moved on, but not before I plowed through stacks of records that were appalling in places. My task was greatly facilitated by Dr. Charles Mullins, whom Ralph had made Medical Director and who had been preparing just such a dossier on his own.

Dr. Mullins became Parkland's first physician president. He left after a couple of years to become the Vice Chancellor of Medical Affairs of the University of Texas system, succeeded by Dr. Ron Anderson, a second physician and Ralph's protégé. Parkland had outstanding leadership under Ron's direction for many years.

The other major contentious area involved the Presbyterian Hospital of Dallas (PHD). Conceived nobly as a private university hospital for the faculty and its patients, it was originally to be located on the medical school campus, along with Parkland and Children's Medical Center. The plan also included a new Dallas Veteran's Administration Hospital (VAH). How splendid it all could have been, but politics soon eliminated the VAH, which stayed at Lisbon, about 15 miles south of the medical school. Then various pressures and considerations led to PHD locating in North Dallas at its present location on Walnut Hill Lane. There was concern on the part of its leaders that private patients would be averse to the Parkland-Medical School campus, and there was the desire to locate PHD close to its anticipated North Dallas clientele. These were legitimate considerations, though the later successful development of private patient facilities on the campus proved them wrong.

Unfortunately, the decision to build PHD in North Dallas, about 10 miles from the school, did not alter the Presbyterian leaders' expectations that it would be the University Hospital, staffed by medical school faculty. Protracted and invidious rancor ensued. A contract was drawn up, specifying that Southwestern Medical School physicians would serve as chiefs of service. Many medical school leaders objected, saying they had not had a say in the decision, and a split occurred. The Department of Surgery, led by the formidable Tom Shires, Jr., had thoroughly committed to the move. When Internal Medicine and other departments dug in their heels, Shires summarily pulled up stakes and moved to Seattle, taking most of his department with him.

As for the rest of the PHD medical staff, the doctors were all to come from the full-time faculty as well as the "clinical" faculty, i.e., town volunteers with faculty titles, thus to constitute, ab initio, a cadre of physicians of more or less proven repute and ability. As the drama played out, nothing of the sort happened. The concept of a highly restricted medical staff collapsed when few of the select doctors admitted their patients, and the elegant new hospital was nearly empty for a few months. The remarkable fresh nursing staff, many recruited at great expense from England and Ireland, was nearly idle. Realizing the error, the PHD leaders lifted the restrictions, and the hospital began to fill.

For a couple of decades, the major departments -- Medicine, Surgery, OB-GYN, and Psychiatry -- had chairmen with tenured faculty appointments. Eventually this, too, fell apart.

ALBERT D. ROBERTS, MD

The Medical School-PHD relationship, along with Parkland, Children's Medical Center, and the VAH, fell in my portfolio. This required me to meet regularly with PHD President Rod Bell, whom I had previously encountered when I, as a witless second-year student trying to earn a few extra bucks as a ward secretary, had donned a nurse's scrub dress, not knowing what it was.

Rod had grown immense by the mid-'70s. About 6'4," he looked to weigh well over 300 pounds. A capable administrator and a fierce advocate for his domain, I found him at times difficult. We conducted much of our business at breakfast or lunch, often tête à tête, at which times his particular mix of crudeness and guile could prove distracting – part of his method, no doubt.

These areas of conflict smoldered for several years without notable progress. The resolution, the dénouement, was rather swift when it arrived. I determined to review the contract, and lo, none could be found. Rod Bell didn't have one. Charlie Sprague didn't have one. Eventually I extracted one from the byzantine archives of the University of Texas at Austin and found that it had never been signed, which meant there was no binding contract.

After that, everyone got down off his stilts, and we eventually went our separate ways. PHD is now the flagship of an extensive network providing care for tens of thousands of patients.

The next decade or so at the medical school involved ongoing interactions with our teaching hospitals and later, some extensive facility planning. There was a crisis at Veteran's Hospital, and an incompetent administrator had to be removed. I vividly recall an unrehearsed good cop-bad cop scene at a meeting of the Dean's VA Committee.

Dean Bonte verbally eviscerated the hapless VAH Chief, followed by Dr. Seldin, whose smooth mollifying phrases dressed the wounds, so to speak, permitting the victim's withdrawal with a remnant of dignity.

For several years, we unsuccessfully attempted to recruit a new Chairman of Psychiatry. The '70s and '80s were low ebb for psychiatry and its practitioners. Much of the patient care had been siphoned off by non-MD's, psychologists and psychiatric social workers. The discipline was having an identity crisis, estranged from the medical model, but having nowhere else to go. By the late '80s, recovery was under way, propelled by the advent of potent drugs and new, more plausible scientific underpinnings. However, in the two decades before the resurgence, many department chairs were empty, many departments feeble, and the pool of candidates shallow.

Dr. Bonte and I almost succeeded in recruiting the young, vigorous Dr. Roger Myer from Harvard and the McClean Hospital. The deal hung on developing a working relationship with the Dallas County Mental Health, Mental Rehabilitation Center (MHMR), and the government-funded organization responsible for providing low-cost mental health services. At the time, there existed a harsh enmity between the medical school and MHMR. Our perception was that MHMR took the money, had endless meetings, saw a few confused teenagers and sad mothers and dumped the truly sick patients on Parkland.

A decisive moment came during a meeting when our Acting Chairman of Psychiatry, Dr. Bill DeLoache, confronted the MHMR Board and its Director. DeLoache broached the topic of MHMR's contractual obligation to provide emergency services. Initially, the Director insisted that MHMR was providing the services, but after a series of insistent, probing questions by Dr. DeLoache, it emerged that the MHMR Emergency Service consisted of the Parkland Hospital Emergency Room telephone number. Bill DeLoache told me the MHMR Clinic displayed a sign reading: "Emergency, 9-5."

The Director was fired immediately, and the MHMR Board members resigned. This was the situation when Dr. Myer, Dr. Bonte and I attempted, in a series of meetings with a reconstituted Board, to build an amiable working relationship. We failed, and Dr. Myer remained in Boston, but this story has a happy conclusion. One Friday afternoon, Dr. Sprague called and asked if I would meet with a New York psychoanalyst, a walk-on who was interested in the job. No one else from administration was available on Saturday morning, so it was I who breakfasted with Dr. Kenneth Altshuler, and the long transformation of the Department of Psychiatry into one of the stronger ones in the county began.

This fortuitous encounter ended eight years' fruitless recruiting efforts, eight years of Bill DeLoache's selfless acting chairmanship. Ken Altschuler had not been on the candidate list because most of his published research was on the effects of early childhood deafness on mental development, a literature unknown to the search committee, and he had only recently emerged as a leader in the New York

Psychoanalytic School. Ken succeeded where we had all previously failed. His smooth conciliatory, non-confrontational style and his patience healed the wounds and ended the conflicts.

The major part of my portfolio was excised in the early '80s when Dr. Charles Mullins was given the job of Medical Director of Parkland and Associate Dean for Clinical Affairs at Parkland. My title changed to Associate Dean – without modifier. This sounded like a promotion, but in fact my role was much diminished. I almost resigned – and probably should have – but Dr. Sprague and Dr. Bonte wanted me to stay on, and I agreed to do so. In fact, I had a few more contributions to make.

First was planning the new outpatient clinic for private patients, what would become the James W. Aston Ambulatory Care Clinic. There is an enormous contrast between what exists now and the situation as it was in the '70s when the concept of important new facilities for private patients first began to be elaborated. In effect, we had no place designated for private patients. I was one of the few members of the faculty who would see private patients. I treated them either at Parkland or by begging for a slot in the Student Health Service suite, which had only three or four examining rooms and one nurse.

But the lack of facilities was the least of the problems. As a first order of business, faculty opposition, based on attitudes, perceptions and traditions, had to be confronted and mollified. That took over a year, and I was the point man with Dr. Sprague's and Dr. Bonte's support. When Dr. Sprague announced the plans to the assembled department chairmen, reactions ranged from dismay to unconcealed rage. Dr. Paul MacDonald, Chief of OB-GYN, went livid, tightly rolled up the printed proposal and loudly whacked the table. This was not the universal reaction. Some departments, such Ophthalmology and Urology, were losing charity patients due to the choices provided by Medicare, and they were desperate for access to private patients. But the weighty departments, such as Internal Medicine and OB-GYN, as well as some surgeons, were initially opposed. Many faculty members regarded private patients as a nuisance. Some found the very idea to be immoral – after all, we were partially salaried by the State, and our mission was to treat indigent patients, teach students and do research. Only a few of us could see beyond this Holy Trinity to what lay in the future. Today at least half the medical school's income comes from patient care, much of it private.

Opposition was systemic and fierce. I spent about a year interviewing faculty members, partly to estimate the resources, such as space, equipment and personnel that would be required, but also in hopes of developing additional support. Dr. Sprague and the University of Texas Board of Regents were going to make it happen, regardless of faculty traditions and attitudes, but by the time construction started several years later, reality had begun to assert itself. A few powerful leaders, notably Dr. Donald Seldin, the legendary Chairman of Internal Medicine, were supportive, and opposition had dwindled to a few pockets of passive resistance.

Two more obstacles remained in the path of developing private patient facilities. One was "town" opposition; the other was the Byzantine approval process. Federal law had mandated that the construction of almost all medical facilities above the level of small clinics first be approved by regional boards consisting of 15 or 20 individuals, only a few of whom knew anything about health care, assisted by a large staff. The purpose was to constrain the spread of new facilities and thereby control costs; enforcement was through the approval or denial of Medicare payments. Pounds of documentation were required to justify any project, as well as persuasive arguments. I was responsible for assembling much of the data and writing many of the arguments for justification. I don't recall personally presenting our material -- Dr. Sprague was superb at that -- but I do recall that the worst migraine I have ever had began as I was driving myself to one of those meetings. When the throbbing pain started, I went half-blind. I dashed into a filling station and downed two extra-strength BC Powders in a Coke. By the time the meeting convened, I was better than normal.

The approvals process delayed the start of both the Aston Center and the Zale Lipshy University Hospital by more than a year. This was a year during which construction costs rose and interest on carrying charges piled up.

Opposition from the large private hospitals and from practicing physicians was more vocal than substantive. One heard of efforts to bring pressure on the State Legislature to cut the School's budget. The physicians, administrators, and Board members clustered about Baylor Hospital and Presbyterian, feeling threatened by the specter of competition from a government-funded institution that, after all, was supposed to train physicians, treat charity patients and do research, not compete for private patients. This reaction, while not unreasonable, was not sustainable, owing mainly to the limited size of the planned facilities, which constituted only a tiny fraction of those in the region.

There was also the argument from necessity. Private patients were needed to enhance learning experiences and to forge quality programs in an environment where few amenities had accompanied the otherwise generally high level of patient care and demonstrably favorable outcomes.

So the new facilities were built, and there was plenty of work for the medical community in Dallas County -- too much, in many specialties. In fact, by means of aggressive outreach satellite programs and successful branding through large-budget advertising programs and generally high-quality professional services, the large hospital agglomerations now command a much larger proportion of the patient population, compared to UT Southwestern, than formerly.

There is one historical aspect of the planning of the Aston Center that should not be forgotten, one that is personally very dear to me. The original Aston Center, known in the planning phase as the Ambulatory Care Teaching Center, or ACTC, was to be a joint venture with Parkland. The faculty were to see both private and charity patients in the same facility, and students and house staff were to be included. It was a very ambitious and risky concept, but it could have been a national model for such endeavors, anticipating, as it did, the blurring of distinction between private and charity as a result of Medicare and Medicaid. It was an exalted ideal, one that may seem foolish in retrospect, but 30 years ago, the contrast between rich and poor, between the entitled and the marginalized, was not as stark as it has now become. I still believe it was doable and that it would have been great.

It did not happen. Dr. Sprague, Dr. Bonte, and I met with Jack Price and Lee Halford, then the President of the Parkland Board of Managers, for two years of joint planning, culminating in my presenting the concept to the Parkland Board. Without the slightest indication or warning, the Board voted it down. It had clearly decided to do so well in advance. We regarded it as a betrayal. I characterized it as "two years of foreplay and a premature withdrawal." The only good thing that resulted was that it was soon to seal Jack Price's doom: it was a major factor in Ralph Roger's decision to replace him.

My major effort during the latter part of my deanship, early to mid '80s, led to Parkland reimbursing medical subspecialty Fellows. Fellows and fellowships had gradually grown in number and importance over the previous two or three decades to become an indispensable feature of our training and patient care programs. But their status was penumbral. Were they house staff or were they junior faculty? Clearly, they were still in training to become subspecialists in cardiology, gastroenterology, nephrology and so on, but they were also providing significant teaching on the wards and in the clinics and carrying a substantial burden of patient care, often without direct faculty supervision. Their salaries or stipends came mainly from research grants. Since I was an N.I.H. Fellow in Diseases of Metabolism for two years in the 1950s, I could attest to the value of this training. But support from academic funds was unsustainable as the fellowship programs grew in size and importance.

It would not be easy to convince the Parkland Board of Managers and the County Commissioners to pay for another layer of trainees in their fourth or fifth post-graduate year. I elected to amass as much supportive data as possible by analyzing existing programs and conducting surveys of many of the comparable programs in the country. It took a year to complete a 200-page document with tables, graphs and reams of data to support our contention. The report defined the purpose, function and the necessity of fellowship programs and argued for the need to fund them.

The young CEO of Parkland, Ron Anderson, and the Board persuaded the Commissioners.

Then came the patient-dumping scandal. By the mid-80s, there was an increasing problem with hospitals transferring unstable non-paying patients to other hospitals in North Texas. Parkland was the major receptacle. This process endangered patients' lives and even resulted in fatalities. Sensational stories appeared in the media. Acrimonious and inflammatory rhetoric flowed. Dr. Sprague assembled the leading hospitals CEOs or their surrogates for a meeting that I chaired. We worked out the basis for fair and workable regulations, with prominent leadership from Ron Anderson. Those regulations became state law and a model for the nation.

The years 1975-89 were among the busiest in my career. I was active in the American College of Physicians (ACP), the Residency

Review Committee for Internal Medicine, and from 1978-81, the nationally televised PBS medical program "Here's to Your Health."

I succeeded my colleague Bryan Williams as ACP Governor for North Texas, and in 1981, I became a Regent of the College. During my two three-year terms as Regent and then one as Vice Chairman, the college expanded considerably, and it began to morph from a staid, mainly honorific old lodge into a more democratic and socio-politically influential agency. The passage of the years has dimmed the memory of long, dull meetings, travel and hotel rooms, overdone and self-congratulatory banquets featuring dull speeches. Despite this, Diane and I enjoyed the company of many gifted and engaging companions, and we formed warm and enduring friendships. And, the College affords a rich access to national medical matters.

The development of the Medical Knowledge Self-Assessment Program, one of the premier continuing education programs for physicians, greatly strengthened the educational mission of the College. During my tenure we moved from the original Pine Street headquarters to the new, post-modern style (Greek temple on top, but alas, no Pallas Athene) headquarters on the Mall.

Meetings at the Broadmoor and the Four Seasons in Philadelphia Georgetown made up for a lot. Most pleasurable for me were my stints as guest speaker -- ACP representative to Regional Meetings in New Jersey, South Dakota, Alaska, Colorado and Alberta, Canada. One of the grandest gatherings was the Air Force Chapter meeting in Colorado Springs. There were more than 200 in attendance. I drove from Vail through a blizzard to get there. The smallest meeting was in Yankton, South Dakota, with fewer than 20 attendees. I flew there from Des Moines in a small, twin-engine DeHavilland turboprop. The airport was completely deserted, and Air Traffic Control was a windsock. But the terminal was a perfect little Works Progress Administration gem. I hope it hasn't been improved. The one good motel, the Holiday Inn, was full, its parking lot packed with Airstreams bound for Alaska, so my host put me up at the seedy adjacent motel, whose lot was full of Harleys. The sign said, "Rooms $18.95. Truckers Welcome. Hourly Rates Available." I had a surprisingly quiet night in a clean room, and a good time at the meeting, getting out just before a storm closed down the windsock airport for three days.

A LIFETIME IN MEDICINE

As Regent, I championed, and was identified with, two controversial issues. One was the Lewis Thomas Award, which recognized excellence in representing medicine in the popular media. The other was a cinema vérité TV series depicting internists at work.

For several years, The ACP had wanted to add to its list of annual awards a media prize to a person or project that enhanced public knowledge and appreciation of medicine, particularly Internal Medicine. The problem was lack of money. A minimum of $50,000 was needed to sustain it, and other budget priorities took precedence. It was not the media award that was controversial; rather, it was the sponsorship that aroused consternation in Philadelphia. I had procured the grant from Ross Perot through a foundation managed by his sister for the purpose of supporting the widows and orphans of servicemen. Ross has always been a controversial figure. He likes to characterize himself not as the pearl, but as the piece of grit that causes the oyster to make the pearl.

When I, with some pride and copious naiveté, announced my coup, several elders recoiled in horror, some more overtly than others. I particularly recall the reactions of Sam Thier, Dan Federman, Ed Hook and Burr Lewis. Despite the misgivings, the project went forward, but Perot's name appeared nowhere on the award or the program, which did not matter to him.

The College should have been proud of the three awards: the first to its namesake, Lewis Thomas himself, the second, to the equally illustrious Berton Roueche and the third to the producers of "M*A*S*H. After I left the Board of Regents, the Lewis Thomas Award was quietly abandoned without ceremony or thanks to the Perots.

The second controversial project I championed was "Healthscope," a series of informational films sponsored by Upjohn and produced by Alvin Yudkof of Silvermine Productions in New York. We produced a series of 30-minute films depicting real practicing internists interacting with their own patients. The management group was initially chaired by John Sessions of North Carolina, then by me. We produced films on diabetes, hypertension, malignancies, home safety and depression, essentially covering most of the areas of concern to internists and their patients. The most moving one by far was on drug addiction. Alvin Yudkof had the brilliant idea of filming this episode, not in a big inner city locale, but instead in a beautiful, small, picture-postcard New England town. The physician and his patients re-enacted their encounters, in the process making the major points: that addiction is a terrible disease affecting patients and families all across the socioeconomic spectrum, and that addiction wreaks havoc on relationships, finances and health. One particularly compelling scene showed a man in his 30s who had lost everything: job, family, wealth and friends. He was desperate, with nowhere to turn. "Do you have any friends?" asked the doctor. "All my friends are Columbian," came the reply. Viewing it, you wouldn't have guessed it was a re-enactment.

Upjohn made no effort to influence any aspect of the program, mollifying the fears of those Regents who feared commercial contamination. Our purpose was to enhance and increase public awareness and appreciation of Internal Medicine. We hoped for a wide audience, perhaps through public television, and for many physicians to show their films to various community groups. Upjohn contributed over $2 million. Several hundred thousand people saw the films, but we were not successful in marketing them to the much larger potential audience that their quality deserved.

It was a wonderful time for me. I had regular, expense-paid trips to New York, first-class upgrades on Braniff and American Airlines, lodging at the Plaza Athenee (under $200 in those days); a pleasant working relationship with Alvin Yudkof, also with the Upjohn folks and with ACP colleagues on the committee. I loved the creativity.

The controversial part arose from the Regents' fear of being tainted by association with Big Pharma. The project almost never happened, but John Sessions, Executive Vice President Bob Moser and I, along with a few others, were eventually able to persuade enough of the Regents that Upjohn's assurances of a hands-off policy were genuine.

I came away from this episode with an enhanced respect for business, businessmen and the strictures imposed by the realities they face, so unlike the comparatively disembodied deliberations, removed from immediate consequence, that inflame the passions of the governing bodies of honorific and service organizations and the halls of Academe. Such reflections, during one of those all-day meetings at the stately old ACP headquarters on Pine Street, provoked the following bit of irreverence:

The Pine Street Pentathlon
(1) Jumping - to conclusions
(2) Throwing - your weight around
(3) Jockeying - for position
(4) Splitting - hairs
(5) Running - off at the mouth

Although I have somewhat mixed feelings about those 11 years, all in all it was mostly exciting and edifying to be in a position to serve on the national scene. I learned a great deal and perhaps contributed something in my time. That was the decade we greatly enhanced the Washington, D.C. office and strengthened our political influence. We oversaw the design and construction of the new headquarters. I helped to select Bob Moser's successor as Executive Vice President, the vigorous young John Ball. There were among the Governors and Regents I served with many strong personalities and gifted leaders and only a rare dud. Diane and I formed enduring friendships: Ralph and Betty Wallerstein, Ed and Linda Maynard, Larry and Peggy Scherr, Mike and Lynn Bernstein, Willis and Anne Maddrey. I served with three fine Executive Vice Presidents: Ed Rosenow; then Moser and Ball; also some outstanding ACP Presidents, particularly admiring Jim Clifton, Jerry Barondess, Stuart Bondurant, Dan Federman, Saul Farber.

Occasionally I fantasize about the life I might have had if I had plowed a straighter furrow, stayed close to home, developed the best small group practice I could and cultivated the life of the contemplative scholar, writing, teaching and practicing medicine. Perhaps it is that secret self who is writing this memoir, at last.

From 1978 to 1984, I served on the Residency Review Committee for Internal Medicine. The Committee is composed of delegates from the three organizations comprising the Accreditation Committee for Graduate Medical Education (ACGME): the American Medical Association (AMA), the American College of Physicians (ACP); and, from the American Board of Medical Specialties (ABMS), the American Board of Internal Medicine (ABIM). Each group provides four delegates; I was appointed from the AMA through the good offices of Dean Fred Bonte. The group met three times a year, and later, when subspecialty programs began to be evaluated, four times. The AMA ably provided the support staff and all arrangements with no fanfare and almost no credit.

We were not paid, but all expenses were covered and we met in attractive resort areas. My first meeting was at La Jolla, where we spent a memorable evening at the home of David and Ava Carmichael. Over the years, we were in Santa Fe (twice), Carmel, Key West, Vermont, and Jackson Hole. The Jackson Hole episode was notorious because of a rare staff mistake. We were supposed to stay at the glamorous new Rock Resort, Jackson Lake Lodge, but instead we found ourselves at a rundown midtown motel called something like the Jackson Hole Inn. In such dismal surroundings, we finished our work in two days instead of the usual three and then repaired to the Lodge, just opened for the first time, for a day or two of R and R.

One January, we met in New York City. Larry Scherr was chairman that year, and he and Peggy arranged a wonderful evening for us, prime seats for "Amadeus." Afterwards we walked through an inch of fresh powder snow to the Russian Tea Room.

The work was arduous. Each of us received a thick stack of residency programs to be reviewed a couple of weeks in advance. We were responsible for a close examination of the field visitors' reports and a recommendation for approval (with a repeat-visit in one to five years) or probation, or rarely, the death penalty, withdrawal of approval. Problem programs were kept on a short leash and given prescribed corrections with timelines. There were many problematic programs, tending to be inner-city hospitals with mainly -- sometimes exclusively -- foreign medical graduates. Such programs were closely scrutinized with sharp focus on indicators of the quality of teaching and patient care, and importantly on verifying that the Residents were not being exploited.

Initially, physicians selected and trained by the AMA conducted the site visits but as time went by, they were handled more often by laypersons with extensive formal training.

The Residency Review Committees made their decisions on these voluminous and detailed reports. Objectivity was a problem, as well as the extent to which the reports reflected reality. An inferior program might be expert at filling in all the little boxes, whereas a good program might do a poor job at self-reporting or have its case prejudiced by one or two disaffected Residents. In our deliberations, a marginal program might get by with insufficient scrutiny if it came up late in the day; better yet, late in the meeting, rather than early on when minds and knives were fresh and sharp.

One example of problems with perception and objectivity was the internal medicine residency at the Oral Roberts Medical School in Tulsa. This start-up medical school sprang from the brow of Roberts and his millions of contributors, and aroused such deep skepticism on the part of the committee that it sent a special emissary, the distinguished academic leader and former committee member, Saul Farber, to personally evaluate the residency program.

Saul came away rather impressed by the energy and devotion of the mostly born-again faculty, which had resolutely put in place all the requisite components of a proper program, and so it was approved. But the medical school and hospital had little community and essentially no government support and were in competition with existing institutions for money, manpower and patients. Charity was soon exhausted, and after a few years, reality trumped zeal, and it all closed down.

There were some gifted people and some vivid personalities on that committee. Strong wills and developed philosophies produced vigorous debate. Harriet Dustan, a hypertension expert from the Cleveland Clinic, was just going off the committee as I came on. She was lucid and low key, as was gentle, scholarly Ray Pruitt, Dean of the Mayo Clinic Medical School. I remember Ray opening his discussion of a troubled residency by saying, "This program reminds me of something said by Ruskin about Sardinia, namely, that it is easier to deplore than it is to describe."

Ed Hook from Virginia and Tommy Thompson from Tennessee could always be relied on to strike sparks, often off each other. Larry Scherr from New York and Joe Johnson from Michigan provided deep keels to keep the big sails on course.

My last year on the committee was my turn to be chairman, and it was by far the most challenging. That was the year Residency Review Committee for Internal Medicine began to evaluate individually all nine of the subspecialties, Cardiology, Gastroenterology, and so on. It increased the workload tremendously. We added a fourth meeting. In the end, it went reasonably well; a practical template was formed and successfully deployed.

Those six years on the RRC were the most demanding and personally satisfying of my decade or more on the national scene. And Diane and I both feel that they were the most enjoyable as well.

ALBERT D. ROBERTS, MD

The TV Star

In 1978, Dallas journalist and author Lee Cullum called to ask if I would be interested in doing a weekly PBS Medical Program. "Dan Foster, MD" had run successfully for several years and was one of KERA's most popular programs. Dan didn't want to continue, so Lee wanted me to try it. The project had received a large additional grant and was to be offered nationally for the first time. It would be a distraction from my real duties and goals, but it would be a useful national exposure for the Medical School, which would be prominently featured. Dr. Sprague encouraged me to do it. Lee and I both felt that the commitment might be a bit too much for one person in view of the many responsibilities I had. I already had a partner in mind, Dr. Anne Race. Anne, slightly older than I, was a psychiatrist, the wife of a physician and the mother of four (a fifth child had died of leukemia). She had begun medical school in the '40s, married classmate George Race when a second year student, dropped out of medical school for 10 years and had her five children. She came back as a third-year student, when I was an intern, and was assigned to my ward team at Parkland, which is how I met her. Then when she was an intern, I was the Chief Resident and she again found herself on my service, where she was a fine house officer who brought an extra measure of maturity to our team.

Lee agreed that Anne was ideal: a mature woman, psychiatrist, wife and mother, attractive, outgoing and engaging. Anne accepted. We auditioned, and the project was launched. Neither of us could ever learn to talk to the camera, which was a drawback. In order to market the series to PBS stations nationally, KERA management decided to add celebrity hosts. Actor Ossie Davis was particularly effective. Actress and dancer Cyd Charisse hosted two shows. The production staff reported that she had trouble with some of the words. One of our sharpest hosts was actress and dancer Rita Moreno, who was married to a cardiologist.

Anne and I never met any of the hosts, their segments being taped separately, but the program and we basked in their luster. "Here's to Your Health" lasted three years on regularly scheduled programming. We did about 50 shows. At peak over 150 stations carried us, and our PBS ratings were second only to political commentator William F. Buckley.

A LIFETIME IN MEDICINE

Each week we had a different medical expert on the program. The production group met weekly to select topics and potential guests and to discuss program content. There were no rehearsals or scripts. We sat down with our guest and talked while the cameras rolled, typically for about an hour. Then the producers edited the footage down to 25 minutes to fit the format of the 30-minute program. After a dozen or so shows, Anne and I developed a sense of timing and could do a 30-minute show in not much over that.

The guest experts came from all over but many came from our own faculty. Ken Altshuler and John Rush did shows on Psychiatry. Roger Rosenberg did one on seizures; Dan Foster returned to talk about diabetes. The other topics rounded out the spectrum of human health concerns: safety in the home, pediatrics, heart disease and obesity.

We had some famous guests. One was Nobel Laureate Sir Hans Krebs, who had elucidated the Krebs Cycle, a fundamental metabolic process memorized by all medical students. Then there was Dr. Frank Engel, often called the father of psychosomatic medicine, though he disliked that term, preferring "psychobiosocial" medicine, which more clearly encompassed his integration of the physical, mental and socioeconomic factors into an exceptionally rounded conceptual framework. In addition to our TV show, Dr. Engel gave psychiatric Grand Rounds. His topic was the Type A personality: the tense, time-driven, controlling, fatigue-denying person who is at increased risk for heart attacks.

After a half-hour lecture by Dr. Engel, a patient was brought in. The patient was a middle-aged man who had recently suffered a heart attack, and he immediately went on the offensive, attempting to dominate the session. Dr. Engel sat back, playing him like a 100-pound tarpon on a 10-pound line, allowing him to demonstrate perfectly his Type A personality.

In the course of this brilliant performance, Dr. Engel revealed himself to have many of those attributes, speaking about his work, his research, and his frequent lectures tours. As an example of the Type A's difficulty surrendering control, he cited his own heart attack. Awakening with typical chest pain, he dialed his cardiologist, a close friend whom he called frequently and whose number he knew by heart. Wrong number, twice: the unconscious at work, fearing loss of control.

During the Q and A, a resident asked, "Dr. Engel, you have told us of your Type A tendencies and your heart attack and the death of your twin brother from a heart attack, and yet we see that you teach, do research, treat patients, travel and write extensively. Knowing what you know, why do you do all these things?"

Dr. Engel let that hang in the air for the psychiatrist's ritual three beats, and then shrugged. "Who else could do it so well?"

For Anne and me, it was great fun. We were never real celebrities, but we did commonly get double takes and quizzical looks in public places. Once, on a flight, a man came to my seat and asked for an autograph for his young daughter. Friends and colleagues would compliment us, and although they were usually unable to recall the topic of the program, they would follow up with, "But it was really good." Once a friend recalled being unable to sleep at a motel at 3 a.m. during a pheasant hunt in South Dakota. He turned on the TV, and there I was! Although he couldn't tell me the subject or the guest, he was certain of where he had seen the show.

After three years, the KERA production staff and management tired of the project and probably of Anne and me. The producer, whose name I have forgotten, wanted what remained of the grant money for projects of his own so it ended, leaving me with mixed feelings. My own celebrity had been brief and inglorious, but enjoyable. Although I fantasized about further developing that aspect of my career, I was also aware that the activity was tangential and that I needed to focus on more serious purposes and goals. "Here's to Your Health" had a few years of reruns (no residuals for Anne and me), finally subsiding beneath the threshold of public awareness, forgotten by all but a few.

The Wreck

Sunday, April 1, 1979. We had been to Parents' Day at Vanderbilt. I remember we were pleased with our beautiful daughter and appalled by the gross obesity of the people lined up to cram down vast loads of buffet breakfast at the Holiday Inn.

On the bright, blue Sunday afternoon after our return, I was driving to my office to clear off my desk for the coming week. Going south on the North Dallas Tollway, I became dimly aware of a commotion of honking and shouting from vehicles going north, on the other side of the median. At that instant, from below the dip in the Tollway just south of the Mockingbird Lane exit, appeared a car coming right at me. We closed and collided in a second. I slammed the brakes and jerked the wheel to the right while he came on straight ahead. Our cars met, our left headlights crashing into each other. This may have saved our lives, for much of the energy of the impact was absorbed by the cars doing a 180, a half circle around each other. I was in Diane's Volvo wagon; my '78 Alfa Romeo sedan was in the shop for repairs, fortunately.

It all seemed to happen in slow motion, seeing the oncoming car, slamming the brakes, turning the wheel, the car skidding and sliding a few degrees to the right, the front of the Volvo slowly crumpling back towards me. I thought I might die. I was briefly unconscious, then a policeman at my window was asking my name and, "Do you know where you are?" First I said, "North Central Expressway," then corrected myself. Then, pain. Pain in my legs as they removed me from the driver's seat, lowering the seatback and extracting me by the left rear door. I was in and out of consciousness in the ambulance, which I shared with my assailant, who looked goofy, unconscious there on the other side of the compartment, facing me, bleeding copiously from a head wound, cheap toupee awry.

In the Baylor Hospital Emergency Room, where I was a familiar figure, I asked the nurses to get a blood alcohol level on him, but still intermittently unconscious, I did not think to order a drug screen. His alcohol level was zero.

I had lost a lot of blood from my fractured knees. I was grateful to see Diane appear at my side, our close friend Pam Mitchell with her. It was terrible for Diane, but seeing I had no head injury was a tremendous relief.

Dan Loyd, the orthopedist on call for my classmate and favorite bone doctor, John Gunn, proposed to do one knee immediately and the other in a few days.

"Oh no! Do them both now!" I said, which he did, wiring my fractured right patella back together, and on the left, sacrificing a large displaced fragment of the kneecap. The impact had pulverized my right ankle. Dan said it felt like wet oatmeal. He repaired it by casting it first then hand molding it into place while the plaster was still wet. I also had a chip fracture of my left elbow and a large bandolier bruise from my seat belt. One interesting fact emerged. When all the X-rays were done in the E.R., Dan asked me during one of my waking moments if I knew I had a spondylolisthesis, a slipped disk between the fourth and fifth lumbar vertebrae. Miraculously I did recall that when I was 15, I had sustained the sudden onset of severe low back pain and that my mother (quite characteristically) had sent me to a robust female chiropractor who diagnosed a "slipped disc" and attempted to manipulate it back into place. Remembering this was important because a traumatic "spondylo," a sometimes seat belt injury, would have greatly complicated my management.

The other driver, who was in an older Toyota and not wearing a seat belt, sustained a closed head injury (bruised brain, but no skull fracture). He recovered to what extent I know not. Our attorney, Paul S. Adams, Jr., found us a good plaintiff's attorney. In the discovery process, we learned something about the man. Rather a ne'er-do-well son of a prominent South Texas physician, he had evidence on a CT scan of an old head injury. This fact, obtained informally by me from colleagues in Radiology, affected my decision about whether to go to court.

This man, who had done a U-turn in midday on the southbound side of the North Dallas Tollway and had hit me head on, had one -- perhaps only one -- good thing going at the time of the wreck: he was employed as an insurance agent and hence was well covered. My attorney wanted to sue, but I pictured a jury trial, this unfortunate wretch with a previous head injury, perhaps not fully responsible for his actions, being sued by a successful doctor who looked young for his age (49) and so obviously recovered. We settled for $90,000 after legal fees, about a year's wages at the time.

The detective assigned to the case contacted me a few times in the month that followed. The police were not strongly motivated to pursue the matter, and neither was I, especially when I was told that the man had later been arrested trying to buy Quaaludes from a plain-clothes cop.

I was in the hospital for two weeks and at home another six, my legs in casts. Diane rigged a hospital bed downstairs in the living room. She provided total care, even bedpans, adroitly and cheerfully. I was, by contrast, frequently dour. When the casts came off, things were much better, and resuming swimming was like a miracle, better than faith healing.

A LIFETIME IN MEDICINE

April first has for us three meanings besides April Fool's: the wreck, the anniversary of our first date (1950) and my father's birthday, 1902. I try to remember to buy flowers for the occasion, honoring Diane's selfless, cheerful and efficient management of my convalescence, I with some lingering guilt over my grumpiness, likely depression that flew away the day I could jump in the pool and swim. (Lest I be accused of limning a saccharine saint, let me add that when not long afterwards I spoke of skiing, Diane said, "Fine. When you break your legs, this time you're going to Parkland, and I'm going to Paris!"

Return to Private Practice: 1983 - 1991

Along 1982-83, I began to think of leaving the school and returning to private practice. I no longer felt that I had anything important to do at the school, and more urgently, I felt that my clinical skills were deteriorating. I still taught both Internal Medicine and Nephrology on the Parkland wards several months throughout the year, but this was not the same as having primary, hands-on responsibility for a large group of patients. Also, I did not have to master and apply the dazzling new technologies; the more-often-than-not dazzling young house staff and young faculty did that for me.

Besides missing private practice, I was also becoming less involved in school affairs. The hospital wars had subsided and planning for the Aston Center was now in others' hands. Half my job evaporated when Charlie Mullins was made Medical Director and Associate Dean for Medical Affairs at Parkland. Kern Wildenthal had succeeded Fred Bonte as Dean. Kern's style was very different from Fred's and I did not feel that I complemented it in the way I had Fred's style. I could continue as Associate Dean for Graduate Medical Education, doing my usual odds and ends and utility infielder stuff that I had always done and rather enjoyed, but my heart was no longer in it.

Kern was very generous, allowing me to segue back into practice over a three-or four-year period. My having kept an escape hatch in case academic administration did not turn out to be a lifetime career facilitated rebuilding my practice. In 1975, I had retained a small practice, about 200 patients, and my partner, Jabez Galt, had allowed me space and staff support in our offices at 3434 Swiss Avenue, near

Baylor Hospital. My talented nurse, Pat Morale, R.N., agreed to work with me the half day a week that I saw private patients in the Swiss Avenue office. I could still admit patients to Baylor, and did so from time to time, during the interval when I was full-time and later part-time at the school.

Back in 1975, I did something I will never live down. I pruned my successful private practice, which had built up to 1,500 or so over 15 years, to around 200.

I composed three letters, each personally signed. One letter stated I was leaving private practice and suggested that my patient seek care elsewhere. The second letter said I as leaving private practice and that the patient might wish to choose one of my partners for ongoing care. The third letter said that my arrangements with the school permitted me to retain a small private practice should the patient choose to remain with me.

I should have known better than to send three different letters going to hundreds of people who knew each other. People in the same office, the same Sunday school class or bridge club, even the same family, received different letters. Dismay and hurt feelings ensued, though people were kind and generous in their conduct toward me. Still, some never forgave me, and I have never really forgiven myself. But in 1975, I was emotionally, physically, and mentally exhausted, and I was not thinking clearly about my relationships nor about others' feelings. I guess it's also fair to plead depression, which caused me to underestimate my importance to others until later, when some told me about it.

By 1988, the Medical School no longer employed me. I had largely rebuilt my private practice with a combination of former patients and many new ones. As before 1975, I was a Clinical Professor of Medicine, a "town man," doing volunteer teaching at Parkland several months a year and teaching at Baylor Hospital. I had a handsome office suite, a competent staff and two excellent partners, Drs. Jabez Galt and Jim Mitlyng, whom I had recruited from the Parkland residency program to replace a previous partner, Jim Borders. Jim had been one of the outstanding Baylor Residents of his decade but had now returned to Lexington, Kentucky, to practice with his twin brother.

Thus ended my second iteration at U.T. Southwestern. An almost complete break from my previous career course, it had enabled Diane and me to live rather large on the national scene through the American College of Physicians, the Residency Review Committee and the two television projects. We developed warm friendships and expanded our horizons through experiences we otherwise might not have had. I had seen academic medicine from near the top, retaining great respect and affection for my colleagues of those years, all the while satisfying myself that that was not what I wanted to do with the rest of my life. I had continued teaching, at which I was good, and sampled academic administration. Ultimately, I was happy to pursue my real strength: direct patient care.

Seduced Again

The return to full time private practice lasted three years. I had no serious thought at that time of ever returning to the Medical School, although I had flippantly commented to Dr. Wildenthal during the final interview that if something good came up, I might return and bring 500 potential donors with me.

It was not seriously said or planned. I was comfortable with my refurbished practice. There were, nonetheless, some areas of concern. During the 13 years (eight full-time, five part-time) that I had been in academic life, my subspecialty, nephrology, had become fully populated by well-trained young doctors specializing solely in kidney disease. Consequently, I was no longer as sought after as a consultant. Hyphenated practices, like "Internal Medicine - Nephrology" had become obsolete.

In addition, I would see more clearly than many where Medicine, particularly primary care, was headed: increasing administrative costs and burdens, lost autonomy and prestige, frustrating complexities and regulations. As each new subspecialty developed, the role of the internist was being eroded and diminished. The Oslerian Model of the thoughtful, humanitarian physician-scholar, competent across the board range of non-surgical, adult professional practice, and preeminent for almost a century was going to be replaced by the harried, necessarily shallow technocrat, rushing through 25, 30 or more office patients, or living in the hospital doing short-term consultative and intensive care, developing no long-term, life-enriching relationships with patients.

I also confess that at 61, I was beginning to wonder how long I would be able to tolerate regular night and weekend calls, so I was not immune to the return of temptation in the large form of Dr. Willis Maddrey.

Willis and I had become friends while serving on the American College of Physicians Board of Regents, finding ourselves allied on most issues and sharing an irreverent sense of humor and a low tolerance for pomposity. He was at that time Chairman of Internal Medicine at the Jefferson Medical College in Philadelphia. Not long after I left the Board of Regents and had been back in private practice for about two years, Willis moved to Dallas to be Vice President for Clinical Affairs at UT Southwestern, a much grander version of the office for which I had originally been recruited in 1975. Foremost among his responsibilities was to rectify the erratic, uneven clinical services while developing efficient access for private patients.

[Here I need to make an important clarification. My criticisms of private patient services are not about the professional management of patients' medical problems, their diagnosis and treatment. By any objective standards, patient care outcomes both at Parkland and its clinics and at the School's private hospital and clinics have always been among the best. In 1990-91, the question was will private, paying patients, who pass by a dozen or 100 competent doctors on their way to our campus, have an experience that will make them want to return and recommend us to family and neighbors?]

The new Zale Lipshy University Hospital had made a good beginning, providing first-rate care in attractive surroundings. In the Aston Center private outpatient clinics, things were not so good. Here and there marginally efficient services existed, one or two equivalent to well-run private clinics. In other departments and their various divisions and sections, fragmentation was a big part of the problem. Attitudes ranged from indifference to outright hostility, not much changed from the Zeitgeist I had encountered more than a decade earlier in helping to plan the Aston Center. Outside of the administration and a few subspecialties, there was still no better than lukewarm acceptance of the need for private patients. Unlike the medical centers at Harvard, Johns Hopkins or Duke, the Aston Center had very few staff members with experience in private practice and scant tradition or culture. The center also lacked any mechanism for effective reform; there was no clearly defined power structure, governance and management.

These attitudes permeated all levels, from house staff to prestigious professors and chairmen. A brilliant young assistant professor in the General Internal Medicine (GIM) division who was admired for his skills reflected the spirit of the times.

One day -- it may have been a Friday -- when everyone in GIM except me wore jeans, I watched the young man saunter across the spacious private clinic waiting area, which was crowded with patients. He was clad in his usual worn jeans, lab coat needing laundering, and tieless, of course. In the middle of the room, with perfect insouciance, he exploded a huge wad of bubblegum all over his face, and then retracted it back into his mouth.

That was it, the spirit: "I'm Parkland, baby, and you're lucky to have me."

All generalizations are suspect, including this one, but this behavior reflects the situation at the time: highly developed medical-scientific skills, sometimes combined with unprofessional behavior, applied in inefficient and uncomfortable surroundings.

Personnel problems were general, systemic and impacted. The GIM division seemed to be a passive repository for the marginally employable. In the academic office, my first three secretaries were, in succession, semiliterate, alcoholic, and furiously confrontational. Firing an employee was no easy task, and in one of those cases, required a grievance-review-hearings process that took many months. Since then I have had good the fortune to work with highly competent and professional secretaries.

In the clinic, my own situation was made tolerable -- and workable – thanks to excellent nurses. As I have noted, my long-time nurse from private practice, Pat Morale, R.N., came with me in '91. When Pat left to pursue a degree in psychiatric social work, she was followed by smart, quick, attractive Dian Melgar, R.N. Dian went on to better things in a couple of years, and then came the brilliant Jeanne Snead, a Senior L.V.N, who had been working the wards at Parkland, where I first encountered her. Jeanne and I worked together until I retired from full-time practice. It is no exaggeration to say that Jeanne is one of the few people on the campus who set the tone for which we all aim.

ALBERT D. ROBERTS, MD

Purgatory

Despite the attraction of the academic environment, the first three or four years after my return to UT Southwestern would have been unbearable, but for the good nurses, In the beginning, I had not realized the extent of the problems, and I misunderstood my role by assuming that I would be able to effect reforms. I was, after all, again a Dean, Associate Dean for Practice Development, reporting to the Executive Vice President for Clinical Affairs. Initially enthusiastic about being able to do what I liked best, patient care and teaching in an academic environment while being an agent for vital reforms, I soon felt frustrated and marginalized. I had no meaningful place in the power structure and no authority. For example, I was permitted to meet with the architects planning the renovation and addition to the Aston GIM Clinic and, in the course of three hour-long meetings, adumbrated the essentials of a dignified, efficient clinic. The Department Chairman redlined every recommendation, and we ended up with another inefficient, awkward workspace.

It was more than a decade before any comprehensive rectification program was undertaken, and this only because of pressure from community leaders Bill and Gay Solomon, Peter O'Donnell and many others like them. Bill had agreed to lead a massive fundraising campaign with the stipulation that access to diagnostic and treatment facilities be radically improved. The GIM Clinic in the Aston Center was to be the index case, the example. Bill and Gay gave a $10 million endowment, accompanied by energy and relentless pressure. As a result, things improved – remarkably so. But this was not one of those projects with a definitive beginning and end like building a fence or digging a well. It was an ongoing effort like mowing the lawn or tending the garden.

Those early to mid-'90s were the most difficult years of my career, harder than internship or the first decade in private practice. I was again putting in 12 to 14-hour days, trying to do it all: patient care, Parkland Rounds, committees, night calls, and teaching conferences. After a few years of this, I cut back and focused on a single purpose, cultivating my garden. That is, holding on to a practice, by then about 1,200 people, many of whom were not pleased by my return to the Medical School.

Following this decision, my discontents abated. Most of my patients stayed and new ones came.

In the early '90s, I had skirted the near borders of becoming an impaired physician with those long, frustrating days, inadequate recreation, and caffeine abuse -- six, eight portions a day. I kept a jar of instant coffee in my desk and most afternoons would add a heaping teaspoon to the brewed coffee from the clinic pot.

The fatigue took its toll in the form of forgetfulness. Occasionally, I would leave my car with the good valet parking at the Zale Lipshy University Hospital entrance instead of my usual faculty parking slot in the large garage across Harry Hines Boulevard. One afternoon, I crossed over to the faculty garage and found my car missing from the spot where I was certain I had left it. Finding no keys in my pocket, I assumed and distinctly recalled that I had left the keys in the trunk lock when I removed my valise. I concluded that my rare 1986 Mercedes Benz stick shift 300E must have been stolen.

I promptly notified both the campus police and the city police, giving details. Then it hit me. I had left the car with the Zale Lipshy valet. That's why there were no keys in my pocket.

This whiff of paranoia reminded me of my father. I resolved to give up being a change agent. Maybe I have had some effect by example, but mainly any influence I may have had was indirect, through influential patients who applied pressure to the Administration.

Why didn't I leave? For one thing, I felt that the decision to return to the school was too big and had come too late in my career to change. The more important reason was I loved the academic environment, the intellectual stimulation from colleagues, students and House officers. And I liked the secure institutional environment, which provided a regular paycheck, pension plan, health insurance, and malpractice insurance.

From Provider to Consumer

The benefits were decidedly comforting in June of 1994, when I was diagnosed with colon cancer. For several years, I had experienced a little rectal bleeding, which I attributed to hemorrhoids, not worrying about it too much because I'd had a barium enema in '89 or' 90 and a proctoscopy a few years before that and every three or four years since my 40s. There was no family history of cancer. I went to see Phil Huber about the hemorrhoids.

ALBERT D. ROBERTS, MD

The procedure had barely started when I heard words you never want to hear from your doctor: "Uh-oh! That's not a polyp!" Unanesthetized and watching the TV screen, I beheld this ugly growth, a bit over an inch across, ulcerated and bleeding. Afterwards I called Diane and said, "Well, our lives are about to change for a while. I've got a colon cancer."

Tom Shires III, who had a bit of a challenge reconnecting my colon because the cancer was nearer the rectum than had been estimated pre-op, did the surgery at Zale Lipshy. A less audacious surgeon would have done the classical abdominoperineal resection and permanent colostomy. In the event, I was restored to relatively normal function and made an uneventful recovery, returning to work in about five weeks. Uneventful, that is, until the following January, when I suffered an intestinal obstruction. This was a miserable experience, two days of painful bloat and vomiting at home and another four or five days in the hospital with conservative treatment, nasogastric suction and IV fluids, until finally my temperature, pulse and white blood cell count all shot up and I had to have emergency surgery to save my intestine -- and my life. It was a volvulus, a loop of bowel twisted around an adhesion.

I had not eaten in more than 10 days, and my bowel seemed to me to take forever to wake up and begin peristalsis, permitting the resumption of oral food intake. Finally, TPN (total parenteral nutrition) was begun. I almost immediately felt better. Control studies show little or no benefit from this, but I have seen the same response in patients I have cared for.

I lost about 15 pounds. Diane commented on the loss of muscle mass in arms, shoulders and upper torso. "Great," I thought, "King's X on cholesterol! I'll eat everything I love best."

Numerous friends abetted me in this, to the extent that when I went in for my post-op visit with Dr. Shires, I had regained every lost pound. I especially remember the sight of Iva Hochstim coming up the walkway with a huge prime rib roast and a quart of homemade ice cream. My classmate and neighbor, Donovan Campbell, came from Farmer's Market with a peck of fresh vegetables and a half case of superb French wine from his cellar.

That was January of 1995. Since then I have not been ill nor missed a day of work except for two days in January of 2003, when a persistent respiratory infection required some bed rest. For some years,

A LIFETIME IN MEDICINE

I carried a nasogastric (stomach) tube and a large syringe along on trips abroad, just in case the obstruction recurred.

After nearly half a century at Parkland, 1999 was my last year to make teaching rounds. There were three reasons why I asked to be relieved. One was my back: spinal stenosis, symptomatic for over 20 years, made worse by prolonged standing and walking on hard, flat surfaces. A second reason was the increasing workload in the clinic and my declining stamina. The third and probably the dominant reason was a wish to stop before my faculties declined -- to go out while still near the top of my game. I still miss it very much.

Many old friends who made practice so enjoyable are gone. Stanley Marcus, nearing 95; Morton Sanger also in his 90s, studying the market quotations within hours of his death; his wonderful wife Hortense not long afterward. She was an intellectual and social welfare leader, a founder of the Visiting Nurse Association. Her house was full of books that overflowed from tables and bookcases and rested in great stacks on the floor; it was one of the best places anywhere to talk about literature and life in general.

Another great lady was Lillian Clark, who also was past 90 when she died. Her vast apartment was full of incomparable art, particularly strong on Mondrians. These were rewarding places to make house calls, not that great art, literature or conversation are needed to make house calls worthwhile. I've probably averaged one or two a month throughout a long career. A house call is often the easiest way to handle a problem.

Observing the patient at home and interacting with family can sometimes reveal more than a battery of lab tests and expensive imaging studies, and the patient and family never forget it. Respect and admiration are earned by accurate diagnosis and successful treatment, but a timely house call brings something close to reverence.

A few honors came my way. In 1989, I was made a Master of the American College of Physicians. This came after my service as Governor of North Texas and then as Regent and Vice Chairman of the Board. In 1995, I was honored as Laureate of the Texas Chapter of ACP. I made a brief acceptance speech, having squirmed over the years as others droned on. I simply said that the doctors I most admired were the quiet ones who get up every morning and do the best they can for their patients throughout long careers, and whose reward is the affection of their patients and a satisfying career. "Ten or twelve thousand pretty good 12-hour days," I concluded, "And it is for them that I am accepting the award."

Throughout the '90s, I had thought off and on about retirement. When I returned to the school in '91, I was thinking five, maybe seven, years. As the millennium approached, I was having a better time of it, as well as accumulating a more comfortable level of security and enjoying improved working conditions. I still loved Medicine and studied avidly.

But there is no escaping the inevitable decline in stamina and intellectual vigor that comes with age. There are three stages in the aging doctor's deliberations about retirement. In stage one, around 60 or so, he starts planning, thinking that 65 might be about right. So 65 comes -- too soon -- and Social Security along with it, but he thinks "I'm too young and smart to quit. Besides, we like the money, and my wife doesn't want me underfoot; I think I'll stay on until 70.

At 70, he thinks he can still teach these young whippersnappers a thing or two, and not long after that he comes to work and finds, mystifyingly, that the key to his office doesn't work, and someone has put his office furniture out in the hall. No joke: this very thing has happened to famous doctors.

The point is there are only two doors to retirement. Like driving, you decide to quit or someone will decide for you, absent death or disability.

I have seen too many old doctors who forgot to quit. Consider, for example, the battered car syndrome: Dr. X has all his life loved cars and taken care and pride in his automobiles. One day you see in the doctors' parking lot that Dr. X's Buick is no longer spotless; in fact, it needs its periodic detailing rather badly. Some months go by and dents have appeared, tires are underinflated. In the final stages, and I have seen this more than once, Dr. X cannot navigate the parking lot without bumping into other cars, or the curb, or a gate, and is himself seen inside the hospital corridors, careening along, long after his hospital privileges have been withdrawn.

In this frame of mind, I began in 2003, age 73, to seriously plan my own retirement. As usual, I overdid it. I couldn't just submit a letter of resignation and make an unobtrusive withdrawal. Instead, I spent over a year going over my lists and meticulously attempting to refer each patient to a physician in our group who would be a good fit. I wrote personal letters and had many conversations, determined to atone for my sins and the three notorious letters of 1975. My official retirement date was September 1, 2004, the end of the fiscal year.

There was a gala dinner celebrating the Tom and Jean Walter Distinguished Chair in Internal Medicine in Honor of Dr. Albert Dee Roberts. Tom and Jean and their children and spouses were long-time patients. Tom was one of Ross Perot's inner circle and a standout among many distinguished executives in Perot's remarkable company. He and Jean have been among the School's foremost supporters. Their generosity in making possible this recognition, and Kern Wildenthal's graciousness in approving it, surprised and delighted me. The honor also permitted me to think that my strivings over the years may have been more consequential than I had been prepared to believe.

For several weeks, I worked on my acceptance speech. During a week's stay in Santa Fe with our friend, Marion Turner, I finally finished one night about 10 o'clock, satisfied, only to awake and find it totally inept. So I rewrote it yet again and tucked it away next to my heart on the night of the banquet.

In the end, I never delivered my prepared remarks. After generous remarks by Kern, Tom Walter and Roger Horchow, I stood at the podium and said, "Everything you've heard is true, as far as it goes." I went on to thank everybody who needed to be thanked, and then told the story of a favorite patient, country attorney Wilfred P. James, Esq., who maintained approximately the same weight of 126 pounds his entire adult life. When I commended him on his meticulous habits and self-restraint, he reflected a moment over his 80 years of disciplined living and said, "Sometimes I think I've overdone that."

The evening was one of great warmth and collegiality, over 100 in attendance. At the table were Jean Walter on my left and Senator Kay Bailey Hutchison, glorious in pink, on my right. My brothers came, our 90-plus year old SMU organic chemistry professor, Harold Jeskey, in tow; and of course our own immediate family. I also included six or seven patients who had been with me since the '60s, recognizing them in remarks about the mutual support and satisfaction to be derived from long-term doctor-patient relationships.

In all, it had been like attending my own post-mortem eulogies, only to come back to life afterward. What a letdown! And the same for those celebrants who only came to make sure you've gone.

A few days later, Diane and I left on our retirement trip.

ALBERT D. ROBERTS, MD

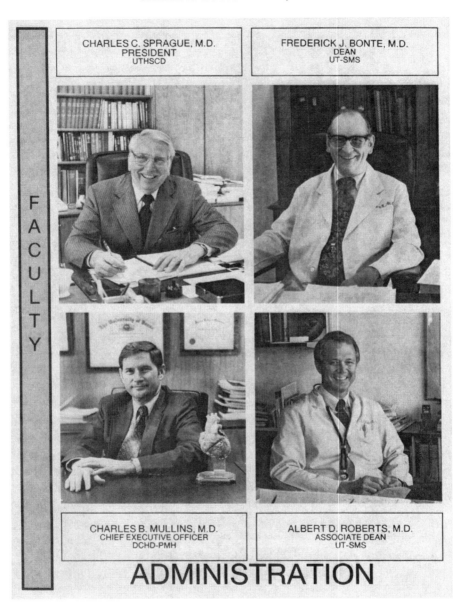

Jolly Adminstrators

A LIFETIME IN MEDICINE

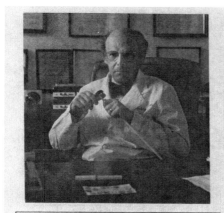

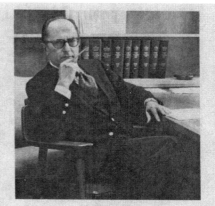

ROGER N. ROSENBERG, M.D.
PROFESSOR AND CHAIRMAN
DEPARTMENT OF NEUROLOGY

DONALD W. SELDIN, M.D.
PROFESSOR AND CHAIRMAN
DEPARTMENT OF INTERNAL MEDICINE

BRUCE D. FALLIS, M.D.
PROFESSOR
DEPARTMENT OF PATHOLOGY

JACK REYNOLDS, M.D.
PROFESSOR AND VICE CHAIRMAN
DEPARTMENT OF RADIOLOGY

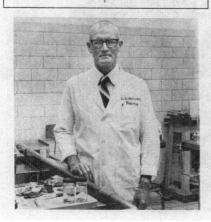

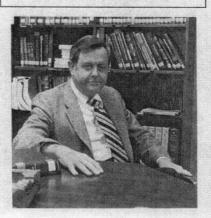

Dour Professors

ALBERT D. ROBERTS, MD

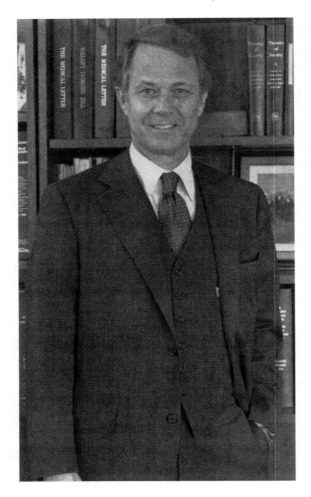

The smiling 45-year-old Associate Dean

Chapter 8

Medicine Then and Now:
An Unbidden and Undelivered
Commencement Address

My father's office was located on the southwest corner of the fourth floor of the Medical Arts Building in downtown Fort Worth. Across the street was a small urban park where we stood in 1936 to watch FDR flash by in an open four-door Packard Phaeton, looking just as he did in the news reels. My father's suite consisted of a neat, small waiting area with a desk for his one assistant and a larger surgery equipped for outpatient operative procedures. His desk and chairs for consultations stood in one corner of the surgery. I remember the white tile, the white enamel cabinets, glass shelves laden with surgical instruments, the bright light over the operating/examining table, the smell of carbolic acid and the sink in the corner. One of my father's sayings in those days – which he denied in later years – was, "There never was a doctor who hadn't pissed in his sink and screwed his nurse."

Next door was the office of Dr. Axtel, a colorectal surgeon in his 60s who wore old-fashioned formal daywear: black cutaway coat, grey and black striped trousers, a wingtip collar and pince-nez spectacles. In my memory, he looks like Uncle Walt's Doc Avery in the long-lived comic strip "Gasoline Alley."

I recall my father describing how the Great Depression created intense rivalries among doctors, who competed for the few paying patients. Some would cross the street to avoid speaking to an enemy. Some carried pistols.

Downtown Dallas also had a splendid Medical Arts Building. When I was in practice there, the older doctors recalled that during the

ALBERT D. ROBERTS, MD

'30s, many practices were so slow that there was illegal gambling in the basement. One of my partners remembered gazing onto Pacific Avenue one hot, torpid August afternoon to observe that there was not a living creature, man, woman or dog, to be seen. Nothing but his office ceiling fan moved all afternoon.

Most doctors managed to earn a living, and although failed practices were common, a good solid practice took six to eight years to build unless you ventured out to underserved rural areas, where you would be worked beyond exhaustion to be paid not at all or with a chicken, eggs, and perhaps a ham.

"Thanks, I'll smoke it later," my father would joke. At the peak of the profession stood a few princely masters of the "carriage trade," free to charge stunning fees.

Such socioeconomic conditions still largely prevailed when I began my medical education in the '50s and persisted until the coming of widespread third-party payers and Medicare.

We were the last of the medieval guild systems. Throughout its long history, the profession of medicine mostly operated independently from judicial and governmental regulation. The traditions and values, the personal conduct and the ethics of the profession were inculcated in the individual and maintained by the profession through its various groups and societies. County medical societies, affiliated with state medical societies and the American Medical Association, had the power to enforce fair and ethical behavior and to discipline errants. Nearly all physicians belonged; their standing in the profession and the community depended upon it. Most importantly, membership was a prerequisite for hospital staff privileges, and staff privileges were highly regulated and restricted.

Physicians could not peddle drugs and devices from their offices. In the 1930s, there was a battle over doctors owning drug stores. In those days, you wrote a prescription, the patient went next door and bought the medicine, and you profited at both ends of the deal. This practice was outlawed to all who desired medical society membership, hospital privileges and the respect and support of fellow physicians.

Advertising was not allowed, and unseemly publicity invited censure, a formal process conducted by the Board of Censors of the local society and voted on by the membership in open assembly. An example of such an event occurred in the 1970s when Dr. Joe Hill, head of the Wadley Foundation, announced a cure for acute leukemia, using a new drug, L-asparaginase.

This was front-page news all over the world, igniting the hopes of desperate parents everywhere. In truth, the child who served as the test case had experienced a worthwhile remission, but not a cure. Dr. Hill was duly censured. The initiation of the censure process required a resolution and at least 10 signatures; I was one of the 10. Soon afterward, I learned that my father-in-law, Fred M. Truett, was on Dr. Hill's Board of Directors. Fred was also President of the Southwestern Drug Company and had led his company to manufacture the new drug. This drug actually has a modest but significant efficacy and has been employed, in drug cocktails with other drugs, for many years in the treatment of acute leukemias. Fred and wife Mayme were angry with me for a while, but eventually understood the basis for the censure and forgave me.

Specialties were relatively few, and they had not yet begun to fragment into today's complex array of sub-specialties.

We had Internal Medicine, Surgery, Pathology, Pediatrics, Obstetrics and Gynecology, Otorhinolaryngology, Ophthalmology, Dermatology -- Syphilology (yes - that's what it was, because the disease syphilis usually begins with skin manifestations and the first visit may be to the Dermatologist); also Neurology, Psychiatry, Urology, Orthopedics. All of these have proliferated into a daunting array of subspecialties.

There were two or three plastic surgeons in the '50s; in Fort Worth, my father was the first in 1946. Few were the subspecialists. In the '50s, Dallas, with a population less than 300,000, had only one doctor, Howard Heyer, who strictly limited himself to Cardiology. He lived well past 90.

There were one or two endocrinologists, a couple of rheumatologists, a small handful of gastroenterologists, two or three thoracic surgeons, same with colorectal surgeons; and two or three allergists.

There were no oncologists. One or two pathologists dabbled, not very effectively in clinical hematology and oncology. Beginning in June of 1960, I was the only practicing nephrologist in North Texas and only the second in the state of Texas.

Nevertheless, from the turn of the 20th century onward, Dallas was distinguished by a cadre of outstanding leaders in their specialties, many of whom had trained abroad before the First World War, typically in Berlin or Vienna. Dallas was fortunate to have had such leaders, men who set high standards of professionalism and quality, unusual in cities of its size, so far from the temples of immaculate learning in, for example, Boston, New York and Baltimore.

That said, until the explosion of sub-specialization that burst onto the scene in parallel with the gathering and ever-accelerating development of new technologies, most of the doctoring was done by general practitioners with only a one-year rotating internship. Incredible as it seems today, a good many had not even had a complete internship. Until the Millis Report was issued in 1966, you could hang out your shingle the day you put M.D. after your name. I had at least one such classmate. My own father, in fact, entered general practice in Fort Worth well before completing his internship. He and others who became surgeons did so by a sort of informal preceptorship, assisting established specialists until the chief of their hospital service deemed them capable of being the lead, or only, surgeon in the operating room. Doctors who didn't care about hospital privileges or county society membership could be whatever they wanted to call themselves.

Registered nurses were nearly all women and white; in fact, white all over: white cap, white shoes and white everything in between. They did not wear slacks or long pants -- dresses or a blouse and skirt only.

The Sisters of Charity at St. Paul's Hospital were an exception in their full-length dark blue habits, topped by huge, stiffly starched winged caps that looked like snowy egrets in flight. Fifty years ago in private hospitals, the nurses stood up when a doctor came on the division and actually accompanied the doctor on his rounds. At Parkland (and presumably at other public hospitals), only Chiefs of Service and senior physicians received such deferential treatment. Now "All changed, changed utterly," in W. B. Yeats' famous phrase. The second of Yeats' propositions, "A terrible beauty is born" is one with which I have a little trouble.

The change in decorum is neither terrible nor beautiful; it simply occurred, accompanied by both improvements and some losses. I miss the formalities in costume and comportment, the refined manners and mutual respect.

A LIFETIME IN MEDICINE

The demographic of medicine is, of course, dramatically altered and would be unrecognizable to my father's generation. Today, women make up at least half the work force, with a large and growing proportion of Southeast Asians, Indians, Chinese, and Middle Easterners. White males are an endangered minority, although no agency has developed to protect us or to retard our decline.

And then the ineluctable drive to specialization and subspecialization, driven as it is by such overwhelming forces: much more money, easier and pleasanter lifestyles (compared to primary care), and the elaboration of ever more complex technology, along with the infinitely expanding consumer demand for the latest and most expensive diagnostic procedures and treatments. Those demands are now commonly created and inflated by the manufacturers, who spend billions advertising directly to consumers and developing special arrangements highly remunerative to physicians whose specialties are empowered to deploy their products.

Few would seriously deny that the accession of women and persons of diverse national origins has been beneficial. For one thing, it is self-evident that the demographics of the medical workforce should reflect the patient population. Cultural and gender diversity in the profession makes for a yeastier mix, hybrid vigor and an array of opportunities for patients of various origins to find medical professionals who speak their language and share their cultural values and attitudes.

It is risky to generalize about women in medicine, although it is commonly done. Do they add a much-needed measure of gentleness and sensitivity? Well, yes, but I've also seen displays of gratuitous toughness and insensitivity, perhaps in reaction to being stereotyped as "the weaker sex" (surely that base canard has decayed in its grave by now).

There is also the "manpower drain" from having a family, and the number who never return to practice or who do so after a lapse of a few, or many years. How this will all balance out remains to be seen. Compared to male doctors of my generation who have had traditional families, women have a handicap: they don't have wives, though some have spouses or partners who share domestic duties. Men like me could work 16-hour days because we came home to a good meal, a well-made bed, clean socks and underwear. I used to compare myself to the picture of Roger Bannister concluding the first four-minute mile and melodramatically collapsing, exhausted, into the waiting arms of his trainer.

One thing is clear: Bubba has had to clean up and compete. I remember the '60s, which crested in medical schools in the early '70s. A few students came to school stinking and barefoot, and some of the females seldom brushed their hair or shaved their legs or underarms.

It wasn't only new competition from diverse racial and ethnic groups that brought about a reversal of those rebellious days. Style's inevitable pendulum would have swung back anyway, but there is no doubt in my mind that the well-dressed, polite young men who wear ties and say "sir" and their equally couth, kempt and courteous female counterparts have done much to set the tone we see today in our medical schools and teaching hospitals.

Previously, I asserted that my father's profession was the last of the medieval guilds. Here I wish to enlarge upon the theme of guilds and of autonomy, its uses and abuses.

Having submitted to the self-prescribed and self-enforced standards of our guild and the State Boards of Medical Examiners, doctors enjoyed a great deal of personal and group autonomy. An individual physician had general authority for the care of his patients. His standing in the community and among his professional peers, and the success of failure of his practice depended upon adherence to accepted practice norms. The contract between patient and doctor was simple and clear: I (the patient) put myself in your (the doctor's) hands and trust you at all times to do your best and to sustain this continuity of care, yourself or your (usually few) surrogates, so long as the contract - the relationship - exists.

This made for strong bonds, essential for favorable outcomes. This earned trust and the anticipation of favorable outcomes, created by the accumulation of many positive outcomes over time, are, even today, the strongest medicine in the doctor's armamentarium. (This is even more important when the actual medicine is weak.)

Honored in memory, increasingly the object of nostalgia, this traditional model of medical practice has now been eroded, almost to extinction, by the fragmentation of responsibility, the burdens of regulation and the incursions of the legal system. The intertwining of the legal and medical systems meant not only more malpractice suits. Thanks to trade law, it also degraded the medical societies' power to regulate physicians' conduct. Nostalgia, yes. Sentimentalization? Perhaps. There is much to be valued in professional autonomy, but it has its limits.

Skeletons in Our Closet: The Downside of Autonomy

"All professions are conspiracies against the laity," quoth George Bernard Shaw, no friend of medicine.

An historical feature of professions is autonomy, and autonomy depends on self-regulation and self-licensure. And self-licensure's felonious cousins are licentiousness and avarice. Unrestrained, doctors in the not too distant past could believe and espouse theories, treatments and operations that seem absurd to us today, but were inflicted on many thousands of victims in past generations, and not necessarily or even primarily by charlatans and quacks. Sometimes such theories and practices came from highly respected physicians and surgeons, including leaders in academic medicine.

Consider for example, the story of Dr. Owen Wangensteen and the notorious gastric freezing machine. Wangensteen, who served as Chairman of the University of Minnesota's Surgery Department from 1930-67, was one of the great surgeons of his era and a leading educator. His dramatic innovation in stomach and duodenal ulcer therapy was to freeze the stomach by inserting a balloon that could be inflated with a sub-freezing solution just long enough and just cold enough to stun, destroy, or at least discourage the acid-producing cells. To ensure precision as to temperature and duration, a sophisticated-looking electronic console was provided. The apparatus was elaborately marketed. Young surgeons around the country were trained in its use, a 1960s prologue to the academic-industrial, drug- and-device consortia that alarm us nowadays.

The gastric freezing bubble burst, along with its subjects' stomachs, which sundered in the dozens. Death, disabilities, and lawsuits followed, and in their wake, damaged careers and tarnished reputations. A model for future biomedical calamity: a powerful and respected leader had an idea; his forcefulness and enthusiasm imbued his disciples with ardor. Criticism and skepticism were muted or abandoned. Industry and advertising seized what was seen as a high road to fame and riches. And then, collapse, at one with the Hindenburg, the Titanic and the Mary Rose disasters.

Such elaborate self-deception on the part of doctors was not necessary in the time before hospital tissue committees, one of the greatest reforms of the past century -- perhaps the greatest single one. No longer is it possible to clip out any organ that meets the criteria of 1) not being immediately necessary to life, 2) susceptible to blame for some otherwise unexplained or vexing symptom complex, and 3) offering a handsome profit to the surgeon. Dozens, or scores, of examples might be cited. While they seem outrageous to us today, in their time, these practices were justified by their perpetrators based on some plausible rationale, current scientific theory or fad.

In fact, physicians and surgeons with distinguished academic credentials have perpetrated some of the worst debasements of medical science. Perhaps the most egregious example in the past century (excluding the hideous but pseudoscientifically sanctioned excesses of Josef Mengele and the Nazi doctors) is the case of Dr. Walter Freeman, the antic lobotomist. A prominent neurologist, he was, at age 40, Chairman of Neurology at George Washington University and a founder of the American Board of Neurology. He was widely published and respected, and one of his core beliefs was that mental illness had a biological basis. Contemptuous of psychological theory and treatments, and burning to find a biological cure, his "eureka" moment arrived when he learned of prefrontal lobotomy. He quickly partnered with a young neurosurgeon, James Watts, and began slicing into people's brains, initially through small burr holes atop the skull. After a few hundred patients, Dr. Watts became alarmed at Freeman's increasing disregard for both science and ethics. Watts decamped, and Dr. Freeman went on to "refine" the operation. A modified ice pick was slipped in above the upper eyelids and jiggled around, severing pathways to the thalamus. The procedure was so quick and simple it could be done in the office. Between 40,000 and 50,000 lobotomies were performed, about 3,500 of them either by Watts and Freeman or by Freeman alone

Many doctors, including some leading neuroscientists at Harvard, Johns Hopkins, and McGill, performed the other 40,000-plus lobotomies. Freeman himself knew that only about a third of his patients improved; most of the others spent the rest of their lives as docile, passive lumps -- but conceivably less vexing to their families and to society than before.

Nonetheless, Freeman's obsession grew as his reputation crashed and his academic appointments dwindled. It is worth noting that it was not the courts, nor the State Licensure Boards, nor even his own victims who rendered him and his operation obsolete. It was the advent of Thorazine in the 1950s. Medication thenceforward offered a more reasonable approach to Dr. Freeman's original objectives, and, unlike surgery, a reversible one, though not without significant side effects. By the time of his death in 1972, Freeman had become the most scorned physician in the world, after Josef Mengele.*

For a third sample, consider the notorious colectomy. It was not long after the general acceptance of the Germ Theory that the theory of autointoxication emerged.

So fashionable was it among the late Victorians that it was inevitable that some audacious surgeon would blame that horrid cesspool, the colon, for half the ills of mankind, chief among them the manifold indignities of aging and senility.

In Great Britain, high colonic irrigation and partial or total colectomy were in fashion. A leading Scottish-born surgeon of the day, William Arbuthnot Lane, was made a Baronet in 1916 for his introduction of an imaginary bowel abnormality called Lane's Kinks, which demanded excision of large segments of the colon in order to preserve the sufferer from the consequences of "stalled stools" and autointoxication.

---

* My discussions of Freeman and Dr. Henry Cotton are largely based on Dr. Sherman Nuland's excellent review in the August 11, 2006 issue of the New York Review of "A Mad House, A Tragic Tale of Megalomania and Modern Medicine" by Andrew Scull, Yale University Press, 360 pages; and "The Lobotomist: A Maverick Medical Genius and His Tragic Quest to Rid the World of Mental Illness," by Jack El-Ha, 362 pages.

Lane did most of his work in London's Guy's Hospital. Many rich, eminent Victorians and Edwardians had their colons and lives truncated and their purses lightened, spending the rest of their days and nights in close proximity to the loo.

A darker chapter in the autointoxication story began when an ambitious young American psychiatrist named Henry Cotton adopted the concept as his own. Cotton was trained at Hopkins under Adolph Meyer, tutored in Munich by German psychiatrist Dr. Emil Kraepelin and his colleague Dr. Alois Alzheimer. Like Freeman, Cotton burned with zeal to find the organic causes of mental disorders and cure them. Being made superintendent of the New Jersey State Hospital in 1907 offered the ideal field of opportunity. He installed operating rooms, X-ray machines and laboratories, enabling the search for the "focal sepsis" popularly believed to be the source of the autointoxication that led to mental disease. Here is Sherman Nuland's synopsis: "He began his crusade with tooth extractions and then proceeded to tonsillectomies, appendectomies, and cutting out the uterine cervix ... he began to excise ever-greater lengths of large intestine because the bowel demonstrably swarms with bacteria."

Fully one third of his patients died. Still, Cotton pressed on, claiming an 85% cure rate. The profession was appalled. An investigation instigated by Cotton's old mentor, Adolph Meyer, confirmed the worst, but Meyer suppressed it. Cotton, autointoxicated by his own theories, "began to resemble his own patients more and more." (Nuland) He died of a heart attack at age 56, disgraced.

Autointoxication has never quite died out. Physicians of my generation (I graduated in 1954) have seen patients who had full mouth dental extractions to relieve arthritis or other ills. There is even a glimmer of scientific respectability: initiation or exacerbation of autoimmune diseases, such as rheumatoid arthritis, spondylitis and Reiter's Syndrome may follow infection, and a relationship between inflammatory bowel disease and arthritis is not disputed, but no meaningful relationship with mental illness is seriously suggested. Nothing can ever excuse such a slaughter of the innocents in the name of science as by the likes of Henry Cotton.

The Greeks thought the uterus was the cause of hysteria in women. (In men, hysteria tended to be ignored, denied, or not considered abnormal.) This calumny persisted well into the 20th century, lightly disguised with a putative medical rationale and bolstered by a surgical "cure" – the hysterectomy. In my own active practice, between 1960 and 2004, I saw many women who had had their uterus removed, some as early as their teenage years, for "female complaints." Anything from painful menstruation to a surfeit of adolescent petulance could provide a basis for removal of the womb.

Since the advent of tissue committees, organ removal must be justified by sufficient abnormality, but still, the organ cannot be completely examined until it has been removed. It is the accreditation process that demands and enforces tissue committees and all the other regulatory mechanisms required of hospitals and physicians by the various Medical Boards, Medicare, and the American Hospital Association.

This casual castration has been virtually eliminated, along with many other operations dear to our surgical forbears. For persistent vague abdominal complaints, there were many appendectomies for "chronic appendicitis," an entity in actuality so rare as to be almost chimeric. If the pain was in the upper abdomen, especially the right upper quadrant, a normal gallbladder might be extracted, leaving the patient with a painful scar, diminished material resources, and the "post-cholecystectomy syndrome"; that is to say, the pain that existed before the surgery, plus the scar.

The kidney was not exempt. For persistent backache, with or without urinary complaints, if the kidney could be shown or suspected to be ptotic (descending downward when standing, a not uncommon anatomic variation in normal, slender people, especially women), a nephropexy was offered. The patient was opened up and the kidney tacked in place. There were few systematic outcome studies in those days, so the possibility that some benefited cannot be ruled out, but the operation is as dead as phlogiston theory.

Outcomes evaluation remains an almost intractable problem in novel surgical and invasive medical procedures. A surgeon has an idea. The procedure is performed on a few dogs or pigs, then some patients. If the patient survives and improvement can be shown, the operation is deemed a success, and it is performed on more patients. The surgeon is handsomely rewarded, since he or she largely sets the fees for the new procedure. Years go by before lasting success or failure can be affirmed, and it shown whether the procedure is better than or even equal to conservative (non-surgical) therapy. For example, it is problematic to know with certainty when or whether back surgery and arthroscopic knee surgery are actually beneficial. A current example of a procedure that is being aggressively marketed procedure by surgeons and manufacturers is the injection of a cement-like substance into the disk or vertebra. Thousands of the procedures have been performed with no controls worth mentioning, and long-term outcomes are as yet unknown.

Invasive medical interventions entail similar issues. It has recently become clear that many patients with stable coronary artery disease do at least as well on medical therapy as from revascularization by means of angioplasty, stents or bypass. Likewise, while electrical cardioversion has yielded some good results in the common abnormal heartbeat, atrial fibrillation, medical treatment, i.e., rate control and anticoagulation, may work as well.

My personal favorite story is that of Dr. Arthur Vineberg, a respected Canadian thoracic surgeon who divined that implanting the internal mammary artery of patients with coronary artery disease directly into the heart muscle would cause new vessels to sprout and nourish the blood-starved myocardium. And it seemed to work -- about 70% of his patients reported fewer anginas and did better on the treadmill. Then some iconoclast did a control study; similar patients were subjected to a sham operation. They did just as well. The control patients were anesthetized and woke up with a nasty scar on their chests, not knowing whether or not they had had the real operation until the study was completed.

This experiment, a paean to the power of the placebo effect, could not get past an institutional review board today. Yet, it illustrates a central conundrum inherent to trying to do control studies on procedures: is it ethical to subject patients to sham (but not risk-free) procedures and deny them the real one?

The thrust to universalize control studies and outcomes analysis can be carried too far. Not every circumstance demands it. When penicillin first appeared in the '40s and was highly effective against pneumonia and gonorrhea, no controls were necessary. Common sense tells us that a new hip is better than perpetual pain and a wheelchair, or that a parachute is better than nothing.

Surgeons are not the only miscreants, merely the most obvious and dramatic. Compared to the transgressions of internists and other nonsurgical specialists, they are low-hanging fruit. The fads, fashions, and rampant "extraordinary popular delusions"* of internists et al are more pernicious and persistent. Invariably festooned with a plausible
and currently fashionable theory, propelled by the passion of the promulgators, bolstered by the ever- reliable and potent placebo effect, and notoriously difficult to disprove, these fad diagnoses and treatments have long lives and wide currency. In my professional lifetime, we have endured epidemic reactive hypoglycemia and "chronic mono" -- two of the most popular. But there have been dozens more around the country. In some communities, the same sort of person

who would have "hypoglycemia" in another area might have "forme fruste" myasthenia gravis, or chronic latent amebiasis. One of Dallas' most respected internists of an earlier generation liked to assign "chronic brucellosis" to the same sort of tired, unhappy, listless people. Epidemic neuromyasthenia preceded the chronic fatigue syndrome.

My own personal experience is that many of these people fall somewhere along the spectrum of somatoform disorders, a group of symptom complexes for which no clear-cut, conventional organic basis can be found.

An intriguing scientific literature is emerging, much in the seven years since I began this memoir. There is often a history of intrauterine post-natal or early childhood trauma that engenders protracted or lifelong susceptibility to a host of miseries, vexing to sufferers and physicians alike. Furthermore, underlying neurohormonal, biochemical and behavioral perturbations are being elucidated. Some influences are genetic, such as mutations in the serotonin transporter gene; others are acquired, for example, alterations in the hypothalamic-pituitary-adrenal axis.

And here's the point: the emergence of a scientific basis for understanding – and explaining – these disorders, accompanied by rational approaches to therapy, renders "fad" concepts and treatments all the more intolerable.

* a bow to Thomas Mackey

The Twilight of Monopoly

The erosion of the more positive qualities of autonomy is being accelerated by a related development: the emergence of novel categories of healthcare professionals to contest the medical profession's authority and dominance. While in many jurisdictions, nurse practitioners and physician assistants are subordinated to physicians by regulatory agencies, the supervision within specified organizational structures is fraying, viz: Wal-Mart clinics staffed by RN's without physician supervision. Such initiatives could be a boon in remote or inner city underserved areas, but the long-term consequences of loose or absent control by fully licensed practitioners are unknown.

Then there are the alternative systems of healing, traditionally antagonistic to orthodox medicine. Not osteopathy, which has been completely co-opted by orthodox medicine. A few chiropractors now function in regular MD orthopedic practices, though most continue to ply their craft independently. Acupuncture has some verifiably beneficial applications, along with a respectable regulatory structure in many states. But there remain naturopaths, nutritionists, health food stores with their resident dispensers of wisdom, numerous varieties of massage therapists, kinesthesiologists, Rolfers; iridologists, aromatologists, and on and on.

In some states, there are recurring outbreaks of pressure by pharmacists and psychologists to be granted prescribing privileges. Among Native American and immigrant populations, there are traditional healers, curanderas, and shamans who are not subject to regulatory standards.

While I don't wish to assert that all such activities are categorically without merit, it is indisputable that the variety of treatments provided by this menagerie of health advisors may result in hazards to the patients, foremost among them: delayed diagnosis, harmful interventions, and adverse interactions between "health foods," "nutriceuticals" and physician-prescribed medicines and treatments.

Physicians, whose medical education lasts 11 to 15 or more years (pre-med, medical school, residency, and subspecialty training), are required to pursue ongoing post-graduate training to maintain licensure. They are also subject to dozens of regulations and are at all times threatened by a rapacious tort system. It is no wonder that they view with dismay this ragtag army of competitors, some of whom have little or no real training nor command any verifiable expertise.

And yet, is it all bad? One can argue that all monopolies are intrinsically pernicious, and orthodox medicine was essentially a monopoly throughout the 20th century, and it retains many monopolistic attributes. Only we, dentists and podiatrists may prescribe narcotics. Perhaps it is not all bad that physicians should encounter competition and be obliged to justify our hereditary prerogatives. Not all of our assumptions are correct, after all. Acupuncture has a real, if limited, role in pain management. Some herbal remedies are beneficial.

Besides, is all our training necessary for the mundane tasks we encounter once we enter practice? When I, for example, entered private practice, I was fully expert at treating diabetic ketoacidosis, had treated dozens of patients during my residency and never lost one. Once in private practice, I saw one or two a decade, at most. What I did see was a steady flow of ordinary everyday minor complaints and illnesses demanding far less training than I had received. Minor acute illnesses and stable chronic conditions are well managed by nurse practitioners and physician assistants, where treatment guidelines are specified and physician supervision is available.

It seems to me that it would be a fine thing if medical practice were to be reconstructed in such a way that instead of graduating more and more physicians – entailing enormous effort and huge expense – we were to train more limited-license practitioners to meet the demands of everyday minor needs. That would free physicians to do the things for which all that training is actually required. The costs of patient care could be controlled or lowered; patients would have quicker access to care; physician extenders would do what they have been trained to do and physicians would have greater satisfaction in applying their unique skills in professional circumstances that optimize their deployment.

The Midas Touch:
How the Golden Age is Claimed by Many Generations of Doctors

In the '60s, when I was a young doctor building my private practice, older doctors of my father's generation would sometimes lay a fatherly hand on my shoulder, look intently into my eyes, and intone, "Son, you'll never know what it was like to practice medicine in the Golden Age."

Then the mid-'60s followed, and with them, Medicare, the rapid proliferation of private health insurance and an explosion of biomedical research made possible by large increases in federal funding through the National Institutes of Health. Physicians my age think it is we who experienced the real "Golden Age of Medicine," certainly the mid-'60s to the '80s, before the nightmare of regulation by third parties stole the piñata. It was a wonderful time to be an internist, when we could practice across the whole spectrum of subspecialties. We were both primary care physicians and consultants, treating heart attacks, complicated diabetes, bleeding ulcers and most illnesses now mainly treated by subspecialists, and making a good living doing it.

Now most physicians 60 or older bemoan the loss of our Golden Age. Many have retired before they intended. "Old boy" conversations at medical meetings and wherever two or more gather are dismal and depressing, more often than not.

But less so if you work at a medical school or a good teaching hospital. The smart young men and women who continue to enroll in our medical schools in plentiful numbers are not in the least dismayed. The challenges they face -- seeing 30 patients a day in the office instead often of 10 or 12? Not a problem. Managing the appalling complexity of dealing with multiple insurance companies? Easily handled by well-trained bookkeepers armed with computer programs.

True, the doctor's office has a completely different feel from the one my peers and I practiced in years ago. Today, physicians usually practice in large groups aided by computers and an ample support staff. I decry the loss of close personal contact and responsibility and the erosion of clinical skills in history-taking, physical diagnosis and the surrender of the individual cerebral cortex to the handheld computer. But I also realize that these young people are preparing to function in a very different world from mine, and they are as dismissive of my generation's dysphoria as I was of those elegant physicians who told me in my '30s that I would never know the Golden Age.

They were wrong. I've tried to imagine the future of the physicians now in their 20s and 30s and I cannot. As Stanley Marcus used to say, the only constant in life is change, and one's only choice is whether or not to embrace it. My experience with young doctors persuades me that they are fully up to their challenges. So long as the core values of this hallowed profession that I have loved these six decades are honored and maintained, the future of those who labor within it, and of those whom it serves, is secure.

Chapter 9

Some Patients Remembered

I am haunted by the ghosts of patients past and passed on. Sometimes these visitations are warm and humorous and sometimes pathetic. A few are painful or tragic. I had wanted to weave them into a single narrative, but found that I couldn't manage the structural complexity entailed. I could well devote an entire book to these honored dead and some still living.

The hardest part is deciding which ones to choose. There are so many who deserve to be remembered. Here are just a few:

James: A Story of Societal Neglect

James was his name. I encountered him for the first time when I was a junior medical student on Pediatrics. James was about 13, and he already had scores of admissions for complications of juvenile diabetes: ketoacidosis, hypoglycemia, infections. As a student, intern, resident and renal fellow, I was to see James many times. He got sicker as time went by and harder to treat because his veins were used up. Inevitably, over the years, complications ensued; impaired vision, failing kidneys, damaged brain. He died sometime in the '60s.

The episodes were sometimes self-induced by failure to take insulin; other times he would have severe hypoglycemic episodes and just go out of control. He taught a generation of young doctors how to treat diabetic ketoacidosis (DKA). I managed dozens of these cases; many were desperately ill, but I only recall one DKA death from those years. That was the one we lost the night we moved to the new Parkland, likely due to a lost lab report. Later, in a busy private practice, with many referrals from other doctors, I saw far fewer DKA's.

The persistent question that arises in these cases is, "Why don't these patients take better care of themselves?" A fellow internist, Dr. Howard McClure, used to shock medical students by telling them, "DKA is a social disease." Howard was right. James and the many like him were victims of poverty, ignorance, neglect, deprivations of all sorts, no social network, and no outpatient follow-up mechanism. These are mostly societal issues. Only the last mentioned – better outpatient follow up – is the business of the healthcare system.

Herbert Hopkins' Heart

Mr. Hopkins began to appear in the E.R., gasping pink frothy sputum, once or twice a week. His sister would bring him. She was a frail little old lady, faded clothes, drooping stockings, sometimes wearing a hat left over from the '20s. Herbert was a ne'er do well who had returned to live with his sister after a lifetime of knocking about. He had been in the Army and received care at the Veteran's Hospital, but his sister preferred to bring him to us for these sudden episodes. So it went like this: Herbert would come in suffering from acute pulmonary edema -- desperately short of breath, lungs bubbling with fluid, heart galloping away. His heart, atypically, was never enlarged, and he responded quickly to conventional care: a little morphine, more oxygen, tourniquets on arms and legs, digitalis. In a few days, he would show up for his appointment at the V.A. clinic, feeling fine, normal-sized heart, lungs clear, and the doctor would stop his treatment, thinking he had been misdiagnosed. A few nights later, the pulmonary edema would return. No one knew about diastolic dysfunction or understood flash pulmonary edema with a small, stiff heart for several more decades, so Dr. Julius Wolfram, Herbert's V.A. doctor, was following the usual practice of the day. Julius was a fine doctor and had a long career in private practice. I lost track of Herbert when I went away to the Army in 1957, but this story has a coda. The sister invited Diane and me to a party; somewhat embarrassed, I declined. I knew that they lived in her large, once imposing, now somewhat derelict house, on Ross Avenue near where the Arts District is now. Sometime later, I related the tale to someone who had attended the party. The guest roster was the Ancient Regime of Dallas, the retired power structure of the city, mayors from the '30s and '40s. Theirs had been a prominent family. I learned she had made her debut in the early 1900s. And we had missed the last of the grand soirees on old Ross Avenue.

A Case of Pneumatic Scrotum

One night, when I was on duty in the E.R., a patient was brought in exhibiting a most amazing phenomenon: generalized subcutaneous emphysema, or air trapped under the skin. Head to toe, his skin felt like Rice Krispies wherever you touched him. But what was most astonishing was his scrotum: the size of a basketball. He had suffered some sort of trauma to the chest wall, a rib or two was fractured, a sharp segment of bone penetrating the lung and into his bronchi. As a result, every time he breathed, he pumped himself up like a blowfish. Inflated, he looked stocky; later, when deflated to his true configuration, he was a thin, elderly man.

Glenna Welsh: A Classic "Teaching Case"

Glenna Welsh was another feature of that decade whom we all got to know well. A slender, small woman with rather nice features, she had the copper-toned pigmentation of Addison's disease (adrenal insufficiency), and she also had insulin-dependent diabetes. Thus, she required both cortisone and insulin, hormones that oppose each other's actions. Too much cortisone deranged her diabetes, but an increase in insulin --one or two units -- resulted in severe hypoglycemia. Lowering the cortisone dose led to problems with Addison's: extreme weakness, very low blood pressure, rising blood potassium, falling serum sodium. It seemed to me that the only times Glenna felt at all well was when she was passing through "normal" on her way to one extreme or the other. She was in the hospital much of the time, this little tan lady, walking the halls. She always had the same response to, "How are you, Glenna?" The small features would pucker, eyebrows up, mouth poised between smile and frown, and a pitiful little voice would answer, "Better?" -- At once a statement and a question.

We student doctors owe a great deal to Glenna and people like her. To have managed her care -- or struggled to do so -- under the severe tutelage of professors like Don Seldin and Leonard Madison, was a learning experience that would be hard to duplicate.

ALBERT D. ROBERTS, MD

A Retrospective Diagnosis

This was a white man in his 50s. His symptoms and signs were episodes of wheezing and diarrhea, enlarged liver, a loud heart murmur and darkened, and irregularly pigmented skin. His attacks were frightening to watch and terrifying for him.

We had absolutely no clue, none of us. The needle biopsy of the liver was not yet being done. We might have considered an open liver biopsy, which would have given us the diagnosis. But the patient had had enough of us. He had been in the hospital a week or so, we had done nothing for him, and were clearly baffled, and every time we poked his liver, he had a spell. So he left.

If only I had saved some of his blood for future analysis. If only I had frozen some of his plasma -- we certainly had drawn plenty of it. We could have diagnosed in retrospect this classic case of the malignant carcinoid syndrome. At about this time, Sydney Udenfried and his colleagues at the National Institutes of Health were working out the biochemical basis of this serotonin-producing tumor. When the work was published after our patient was "lost to follow-up," I realized what we had missed. The unfortunate patient had not long to live, with or without a diagnosis, and 50 years later we still don't have a satisfactory treatment.

Wilfred P. James, Esq.: Elegant Small-Town Lawyer

Wilfred P. James, Esq. was about 80 when I met him. He had come to Dallas from his home in East Texas for eye surgery in the old Medical Arts Building. His ophthalmologist referred him to us for a pre-op check-up; my partners were too busy, so I saw him, and a friendship began.

Mr. James was elegantly old-fashioned. Tall and very slim, he always wore a three-piece black suit, white shirt, thin black tie, gold watch chain draped on the vest, a wide-brimmed, soft-crowned black hat, and, of course, shiny black shoes and black knee-length stockings secured by garters. Then picture a small, well-shaped head, neatly trimmed white hair, blue eyes behind gold-rimmed spectacles, and you have Mr. James. I always imagined him as the elderly bachelor cousin or brother of William Faulkner's country attorney, Gavin Stephens. He was maybe the last man to wear one-piece cambric underwear and rice powder.

Still active in his law practice with his nephew (also a patient of mine, colorful in different ways), Mr. James was proud of the fact that he and his deceased brother had tried at least one case in every one of Texas' 254 county courthouses.

He was soft-spoken and quietly humorous in a quizzical sort of way. I always looked forward to his two-or three-times a year visits and was proud to be his internist.

One day, standing on my examining-room scales, he peered intently at the numbers and asked, "How much do I weigh?"

"Mr. James, you weigh 126 pounds."

"I've weighed 126 since my 20s," he said. "What do you think about that?"

"Mr. James, I'd say that means you are a man of very meticulous habits."

Wilfred P. James, Esq., in his one-piece cambric underwear, looked back over the nearly 60 years, then said, "Sometimes I think I've overdone that."

He died peacefully in his sleep a year or two after that. I learned this from his nephew and law partner, Larry James, who was opposite to Wilfred as he could be. Larry loved Luckies, bourbon and SMU. Bad habits clogged up his arteries. His first symptom was that his watch, which he wore on the left wrist, ran down. His subsequent stroke was left-sided, when his right middle cerebral artery thrombosed.

Ondine's Curse

She was a trim, intelligent brunette in her late 40s who was working as a secretary. Her complaint was headache -- a severe, throbbing headache that came on at night and responded poorly to aspirin or Tylenol. She had a poignant and appalling history: diagnosed with advanced pulmonary tuberculosis in her late 20s, before antibiotics, she had spent eight years in a sanitarium. The infection had finally been controlled, conceivably cured, though it was hard to tell with such extensive scarring. Then, she had just begun to assemble a normal life for herself when she developed cancer in both breasts. She had had bilateral radical mastectomies followed by irradiation, which likely further scarred her lungs. This sequence had been completed two or three years before I saw her and listened with dismay to her story.

When I saw her chest X-rays, I could scarcely believe that she could be out of bed, let alone working, and not even be short of breath.

A further shock came when I examined her retinae: the ophthalmoscope revealed hemorrhage, exudates and papilledema (swelling of the optic nerve at its entry into the retina), changes seen in malignant hypertension, brain tumors and other causes of elevated intracranial pressure. Yet, she had normal blood pressure and no abnormal neurological findings on examination. Suspecting a brain tumor, I referred Virginia to a neurosurgeon to perform bilateral carotid arteriograms. (Radiologists did not yet do the procedure, and CT scans and MRIs were decades in the future). A brief period of general anesthetic was administered. Virginia did not wake up from the anesthetic and appeared to have stopped breathing. I got a panicky call from the neurosurgeon and dashed down to X-ray, where I found my patient unconscious, purple and not breathing. I called her name and shook her, and she opened her eyes and started to breathe; in a little while, she returned to her usual state.

The carotid arteriogram was negative. The arterial pattern disclosed no deviation from normal as would be seen by any space-occupying lesion.

At this point, comprehension glimmered. I was aware that both carbon dioxide retention and low blood oxygen levels could cause elevated intracranial pressure (pseudo tumor cerebri, or idiopathic intracranial hypertension). I just had not previously suspected this situation in Virginia's case. She was not breathless or cyanotic, and the one set of blood chemistries that I had done had shown a bicarbonate (CO_2) level barely above normal, not enough to excite my suspicions. Arterial blood gas measurements, the gold standard for oxygenation problems, have been a routine procedure for decades now, but in the '60s, it was only occasionally done by special order. When Virginia's arterial blood gases were measured, the levels were so abnormal as to be barely compatible with life – and this was 10 or 15 minutes after she started breathing again.

Then I understood. Virginia suffered from Ondine's Curse. In German mythology, Ondine was a beautiful water nymph who surrendered her immortality by marrying a mortal and bearing his son. Sir Lawrence had sworn when they wed that with every waking breath he would think of her. The formerly immortal Ondine aged faster than her handsome knight did. One day finding him in the arms of another woman, she delivered her curse: that he would have to think consciously to breathe, meaning he would die if he fell asleep.

The syndrome was so-named by Severinghaus and Mitchell in 1962 in a paper describing three patients who developed the central alveolar hypoventilation syndrome in association with high brainstem surgery. It was subsequently described in pregnancy, in severe mechanical disturbances of respiration and as congenital failure of the respiratory center to develop.

Virginia's respiratory center had become insensitive to the stimuli to respiration, a rising blood bicarbonate (CO_2) or, to a lesser extent, a falling blood oxygen. There was probably an initial physiological tradeoff: accepting the abnormal levels ameliorated the work of breathing, moving air in and out of her rigid chest and scarred lungs.

For Virginia, the tradeoff had gone too far. When she was awake and active, her respirations were marginally adequate. When she slept, her breathing almost ceased, her oxygen levels plummeted, bicarbonate levels soared precipitously, causing a rise in intracranial pressure, which resulted in a throbbing headache, which awakened her and kept her from dying in her sleep.

Had we been able to provide her with a chest respirator and low-flow oxygen while sleeping, her decline might have been slowed or arrested, but such means were not yet available. I tried various medications, for example, progesterone, known to stimulate the respiratory center. We tried having her set her alarm clock to go off hourly for some minutes of consciously driven breathing. But the deranged physiology had gone too far, and she gradually declined and died a few months later. I attended her frequently toward the end in her tiny, rented room, barely big enough for a bed. She remains fixed in my memory, one of the most tragic cases and one of the bravest people I have known.

Jesse Walsh's Peaceful Passage

Jesse and her husband Dan were friends of my wife's parents, part of their circle of close friends, all a generation older than Diane and I. Jesse and Dan, who were childless, were considerate and friendly toward us and, in fact, had helped with our wedding and reception. They were landscape architects, both quite talented and artistic, with a wide range of knowledge and interests. Jesse was the more dominant personality; her name suited her somewhat androgynous appearance and character. She was said to have been pretty when young, but in middle age, her face was ravaged by the effects of a lifetime of heavy cigarette smoking. She was too thin, her face not so much wrinkled as corrugated, and she had stained teeth and fingers.

She had, however, great personal style and unerring taste in everything that interested her. She was an expert on all aspects of gardening and landscape, and was also knowledgeable about art, both fine and decorative, as well as antiques, American, European and especially Chinese.

She wore fashionable clothes with easy grace, and she was a pleasant conversationalist and an easy dinner companion.

Jesse had been raised a Christian Scientist, and she remained mostly true to the teachings. Yet she wanted me to be her doctor, and this presented obvious difficulties. Having never sought medical treatment, in her 60s she began to think that she might need a doctor, but she had no idea how to interact with the medical profession, nor did her husband, who was not a Christian Scientist. He had just rarely been sick or been to a doctor. During her office visit, Jesse had some difficulty describing her health concerns. She reluctantly permitted a limited physical examination, a chest X-ray and some simple lab tests.

And this may have been all I needed to guess how things would go. The chest X-ray showed scarring and emphysema, though not as bad as I expected, but no cancer or infection. And there were no palpable masses anywhere. Being so thin, she was easy to examine, as far as I was allowed, but no pelvic.

What was readily apparent was the extensive arterial disease. The heavy smoking had ruined her circulation; her arteries were like pipe stems, loud murmurs over her neck, chest, abdomen and groin, and the chest X-ray had revealed calcium deposits lining the arteries – almost more calcium in the aorta than in the vertebrae.

In any case, these were all the findings that I was to have except for ongoing observation. Dan and I watched while Jesse dwindled. There was not a bit of pain, little if any discernible mental decline. She wasted away before our eyes, almost certainly from mesenteric vascular insufficiency: the partially blocked arteries to her digestive system precluded adequate absorption of nutrients. In effect, she starved to death over a period of months. The last few weeks, she could scarcely rise from bed and required 24-hour nursing attendance. Dan, whose comprehension of these events was fairly limited, called daily, and I went by frequently with nothing to offer except sympathy and support.

One evening Dan called and from what he related, I thought Jesse was at last on her way out. I sat with Dan and the nurse for about two hours while what remained of Jesse quietly, gradually, stopped breathing.

In over a half century in medicine, it was the only completely natural death I have ever simply watched: no tubes, no machines, no bright lights or cold steel, at home in her own bed, no medical interventions of any kind. It was beautiful.

That was over 30 years ago. Even today, with modern surgery and arterial stenting, I doubt her life could have been prolonged in any satisfactory way.

This account is certainly not an argument for Christian Science, which did not save her from chronic nicotine poisoning, and she was lucky not to have suffered from some of its more painful – and more common – consequences. Still, I have to admit, in some ways, her faith served her rather well.

As a coda, I will add that the few other Christian Scientists I have had as patients have also been easy to deal with, because they expect so little from their (terrestrial) doctor.

Eleanor Price

She was 16, a fine-looking young woman with a beautiful, fully formed figure. Her father had recently died of a malignancy under the care of one of my partners. Eleanor and her mother became patients of mine. We met for the first time as doctor and patient in the Presbyterian Hospital Emergency Room where Eleanor, almost comatose and in critical condition had been brought by her anxious mother. It was clear that Eleanor was in diabetic coma – ketoacidosis, far advanced. She had no previous history diabetes and neither parent was diabetic.

As bad as it was, the ketoacidosis was not the worst of it. Here, the worst thing was the infection that precipitated the DKA: Eleanor had fulminant genital herpes. Her first sexual encounter was devastatingly unlucky. The entire perineum and vaginal mucosa were covered with painful blisters. She was in agony, in addition to being critically ill with new onset DKA. Herpes can become generalized and life threatening in immunocompromised states, which include uncontrolled diabetes.

But she was young and fundamentally strong. She responded quickly to conventional treatment for the DKA – proper fluid replacement; careful insulin dosing – and the herpes followed the normal course, crusting over and healing in about six weeks. As I have observed in other patients who suffer from herpes, have strong immune systems and suffer a violent first attack, she never, to my recollection, had another attack of herpes.

Nor, happily, of ketoacidosis. But she was a juvenile-type diabetic, and not one of the lucky ones who magically escaped the complications for decades. Eleanor had a decade or so of a normal existence except for the demands of her labile diabetes, with its ups and downs and constant daily need for attention to diet, level of activity and insulin dosage. She was a good patient who managed things very well and never had serious trouble with her blood sugar. She married a promising young man, and things went well for several years. Then her husband was killed in an automobile accident.

By the time she was 30, the complications began to creep in: a bit of protein in the urine, a little rise in blood pressure, slight decline in kidney function, and telltale "berry" aneurysms in the retinas.

For 10 or 15 more years, she had few troublesome symptoms. The eye complications were well managed by the ophthalmologists. The decay in cardiovascular and kidney function proceeded implacably but not so perceptibly (to her) until compensatory reserves and mechanisms were finally overwhelmed by disease progression.

For much of this interval of quiet disease progression, she was not under my care, owing to her HMO – I was not in her network. Also during this interval she remarried – a kind, humorous, sturdy fireman whom I immediately liked and who was totally devoted to Eleanor.

Eleanor returned to my care about the time I returned to the medical school for the second time in 1991. By then, the complications were well advanced. Her kidneys had failed, and she was in regular hemodialysis. She had suffered heart attacks. There was a long bout with eye inflammation that would have cost her eyesight but was eventually controlled by strong immunosuppressive drugs (cyclosporine and prednisone). She developed severe arthritis of a peculiar type that occasionally afflicts diabetics. It is not so much joint

A LIFETIME IN MEDICINE

inflammation as a severe thickening of tendons, joint surfaces and soft tissues by connective tissue proliferation; this process particularly affected her hands, wrists, ankles and feet. The entity of nephrogenic systemic fibrosis was described in detail only some years after Eleanor died. In retrospect, this is clearly what happened to her, and was associated more with renal failure than with diabetes.

She never complained, and she continued to function in all her roles and duties, though she worried a bit that she could not really please her husband in bed.

Decline was slow but inexorable. Medically we had at least some kind of answer for every problem, some better than others, but nothing could affect the fundamental progression of her disease.

Eleanor never stopped taking care of her husband until she died. She kept the books, managed the household accounts and the household itself right up to the end. J.B., her husband, dreaded losing her not only because he loved her deeply, but also he was afraid he would be lost without her, in all things great and small. What he dreaded most was the income tax return. He had never done his own, had no idea what you had to do or even where the necessary information was kept, except maybe somewhere in Eleanor's desk.

Sometime a while after April 15th of the year Nancy died; J.B. came for his annual physical and visit. He told me that when he opened Nancy's desk, he found the income tax return completely done. Nancy had died not long after the first of the year. The tax report was her last, posthumous gift to her husband. He cried a little, telling me the story. And I almost did, hearing it.

Hermione Leake

I had a call from patients who lived in an attractive brick house in University Park. The call was about his next-door neighbor, Mrs. Leake. This was in the '60s. The upscale Park Cities (as neighboring Highland Park and University Park are known) still had a few pockets of desolation and despair. Forty years ago the epidemic of ostentatious affluence manifested by the overnight demolition of hovels like Mrs. Leake's and the almost equally abrupt erection of looming, zero-lot-line turreted, rococo mansions had not yet begun.

Even so, the Leake cunabula stood, or more accurately, leaned, in dramatic contrast to the aspiring bungalows on either side, like a beggar at a wedding feast. My patients, who were also friends, were concerned, and not just about appearances: sanitation and property values were at issue. They wanted me to visit their neighbor, which I did.

The house, once a white frame one-story, had not been painted in a generation. The yard was equally untended. Inside, it was even worse. A few pieces of decrepit furniture rested on warped raw wooden floors, on which one stepped vigilantly, owing to the 21 free-ranging cats. The sole inhabitants' housekeeper, a short, muscular black woman of around 40, met me at the door. She had a direct gaze and manner. Her face and arms were covered with scars.

"Knife fights," she explained.

She led me to the bedroom in the back of the house, where I found Mrs. Leakes lying among stained bedclothes, wearing an unclean cotton nightdress. She was in her mid-80s, as disheveled and unkempt as her surroundings. Despite a somewhat wild gaze, she was alert and seemingly in command of her mental faculties.

As is usual with patients who have seldom or never had medical care, obtaining a conventional medical history was not easy. She could not really describe her own condition and struggled to understand my questions, but we got along reasonably well, and she developed a wary confidence in me and permitted a cursory examination, with the black warrior and many cats in attendance.

Her skin was mottled with innumerable purple and black bruises, not wounds, but purpura, skin hemorrhages related to a clotting deficiency, or to senile skin changes and possibly to scurvy (Vitamin C deficiency) and/or inflamed blood vessels. Mrs. Leake had all of these disorders, in fact. There were also open, draining sores on her legs, sores that had never seen a dressing or medication, as a glance at the bed sheets confirmed.

I also was told that the oldest cat was 23.

She reluctantly agreed to come to the office for a few tests. It developed that she had lupus – systemic lupus erythematosus (SLE) and pernicious anemia. We started her on B12, low-dose prednisone, and daily wound dressings. Her attendant was competent and helpful. Our patient rallied and did well for a few months; but then she declined. Just too many years and too many illnesses. I don't recall her actual terminal episode or what happened to the cats and the attendant.

In keeping with the neighborhood, the house was immediately demolished and replaced by a conventional two-story brick house.

Cloyd Fuller

To do justice to Cloyd with any economy of words and without overtaxing my readers' credulity is a challenge. He was in his late 20s the day he first came to my office. He was about 5'8" and 150 pounds, black hair above a low forehead, blue eyes and rather good-looking features. A slender, muscular physique – not from any kind of training, but from good genes and a vigorous life. He wore cheap white shirts and black chinos from Penney's, a good leather belt, and tired Wellington boots. He was the tenth son of a Kansas sharecropper, and he had hundreds of stories to tell. This is how he opened the interview.

"I'm gonna tell you why I don't trust doctors."

He spoke with a real country accent and lots of expression and gesture, a slight sideways gaze until he came to the end of the sentence, which he punctuated with a very direct glance.

"I was real athletic in high school, ran track and played baseball and football. The trouble was, one year someone decided it would be a good idea for all the athletes to have physical examinations. When the doc listened to my heart, he told me I had a real bad heart and could not play sports at all or exert myself.

"My dad took me to a heart specialist in Kansas City. This doctor listened to my chest and made a cardiogram and a chest X-ray. When he came back in carrying the X-rays, he looked very concerned, told me I had something real bad wrong with my heart and needed an operation right away or I might not live long.

"My dad said, 'Well, doc, we're just poor sharecroppers. We don't have no insurance or money or anything.'

"So then the doctor says, 'Well, son, you just go on home and take it real easy, and come back and see me next year'."

"Well shucks," Cloyd went on, "I figured if I was going to die pretty soon, I might as well have a good time, so I started drinking and smoking and chasing girls full-time. I had to have a job to pay for all my bad habits, and I stayed in school, played all the sports same as always and made good grades. I was sleeping about two hours a night and felt fine all the time. I even saved a little money and went back to the heart specialist. He listened to my heart, made a cardiogram and a chest X-ray. When he was through, he came back in and said, 'Son, you sure have been living right!'"

That was how Cloyd introduced himself, and his story told me much of what I needed to know about him – that he was smart, tough, independent, skeptical and given to intemperate habits, at least at times. He was also extremely droll.

When I examined him, I understood the doctor's concern. Cloyd had a Grade VI systolic heart murmur, one you could hear without a stethoscope if you placed your ear an inch or two from the chest wall. The echocardiogram revealed pulmonic stenosis – a tightly narrowed pulmonic valve that he was born with. He was fond of telling the story that he was born a blue baby and that the doctor or mid-wife had ordered him placed in the oven to pink up. Perhaps this story is true, or perhaps it is one of Cloyd's entertainments – though I have no doubt he believes them all to be true – but pulmonic stenosis is not one of the congenital heart diseases that causes cyanosis, i.e. "blue babies."

As often happens, this focus on his heart left Cloyd with a permanent preoccupation with it. He felt every beat and every missed beat and was prey to almost daily pains of his chest, pains he liked to call "indigestion." He lived in a state of apprehension except when he was working or drinking, two activities he pursued energetically. He worked as a contractor, and, as it gradually became clear to me, he was an extremely successful one. He lived in a house he had built on a farm some 20 miles from the city, with his perpetually sick, chain-smoking wife. He raised three sons, all of them college graduates. The drinking could be continuous over time, or else periods of sobriety punctuated by binges, much of it to allay his anxiety. With one exception, he was sober when he came to see me, and he always had a story. Sometimes he would reminisce about the "running drunks" of his youth, four or five buddies in someone's car, driving hundreds of miles – Mexico, Cabo, Louisiana – and staying drunk 'til the money ran out.

One day when we had known each about 30 years, I took him into an examining room and told him I couldn't do anything for him if he didn't stop drinking, and not to come back unless he did quit.

And quit he did. That was some years ago. Subsequently I saw him through a bout of bacterial endocarditis and two bouts of upper gastrointestinal bleeding. But in recent years, he has done well. He has barely enough liver left to get by, but he's active and successful in his work and in his 60s the anxieties have abated.

His wife finally died from consequences of chain-smoking. I think all but one of his brothers are gone, tobacco, alcohol, violence in some cases.

But Cloyd goes on. I have known some prized rednecks in my time. A few of them were pretty mean. Many or most were admirable. Cloyd is the best of the breed. I could write a whole book about him and his stories.

In a Lighter Vein

The practice of medicine is tragic and comic, humiliating and inspiring, and to all who really watch and listen, endlessly instructive. Every day brings challenges. Some are met and overcome but some are not. Some are not even recognized. Others are dodged. With age and maturity, one learns which ones to avoid.

For instance, there was the time the World Championship of Tennis tour came to Dallas. This was a great event, long ago abandoned, that was played in the large enclosed basketball arena on the SMU campus, seating for 8,000. I saw one of the all-time great matches there, Ken Rosewall versus Rod Laver at the peak of their games. Rosewall finally won at the end of five long sets with one of his impossible backhands down the line.

Another year, John Newcombe played a 17-year-old Bjorn Borg in the championship match. At 29, Newcombe was having his best year, and this was probably his last chance to finish number one in professional tennis. But he had a problem: during his previous match, he had suffered severe abdominal cramps. A recurrence might cost him a victory and the title he wanted badly.

My friend and patient, Rip Collins, was one of the promoters of the event. Rip made me a proposition: I would have two prime seats free if I would agree to administer a shot of anesthetic and cortisone into Newcombe's belly muscles if the cramps recurred during the match (After his previous match, Newcombe's complaint had been dramatically relieved by such an injection). Newcombe would send a hand signal, and I would dash down onto the arena floor, kneel down, and, in front of 8,000 people, inject the contents of a large syringe into Newcombe's belly muscles.

Why I agreed to be involved in this is hard for me to explain to myself – let alone excuse – but I was starry-eyed over being a part of the great event, and, doubtlessly foolish. Imagine if Newcombe had convulsed and died right there before 8,000 people, young Dr. Roberts at his side, empty syringe in his hand? Unfortunately, this prospect did not occur to me until I was in my seat watching the match. Luckily, nothing happened. Newcombe won his match and his title, though not easily. Afterward Borg said, "Well, I'm young. I'll be back."

My Most Embarrassing Moments

It was in the early '60s. There I was, a young hotshot former chief resident, well embarked on a successful career. I was performing rigid proctoscopy on a woman in her 30s, her first visit to our office. Some worrisome bowel complaint had prompted the examination. Rigid proctoscopy is seldom performed today, having been replaced by the much more humane flexible scopes that can do the entire colon. In the rigid proctoscopic exam, the patient was placed in the "knee-chest position" either on a conventional examining table with the rear end up almost at eye level, anus exposed while the head and arms were cradled on a pillow. Or else the patient was placed in a similar, jack-knife position on a motorized examining table, an apparatus which we lacked. I made a lame little joke, "We don't usually do this on the first date," and inserted the proctoscope, whereupon, I was shocked and surprised to discover what I had first took to be a large tumor, the size of a small lemon, near the orifice. On closer inspection, I was horrified to observe that the "tumor" was uniform in appearance and contained a small central hole. It was in fact, the cervix, and I had inserted the instrument into the wrong place by mistake. I confessed my error and completed the proper examination, which was negative. The patient was speechless, had a sort of stunned look on her face and hurriedly left. I did not submit a bill, and she never returned. I was lucky, very lucky, that this happened early in my career before the epidemic of litigation began. Any time in the last 20 or 30 years, I would have been sued for all I possessed.

In another case, a particularly good-looking young woman had come for a pelvic examination. She was in the lithotomy position, an archaic term describing the position that patients were placed in for the extraction of bladder stones in the remote past. Her pelvis was unusually capacious, and I was having some difficulty palpating her ovaries. After a while she asked, "Doctor, did you lose something?"

On another occasion, a young woman had brought her mid-50s mother in for her very first complete physical examination. When time came for the pelvic, I explained it as best I could and proceeded as sensitively and carefully as I could, but she tensed and cringed and gradually ooched up toward the head of the table while I attempted to complete at least a minimal examination. Trying to help her relax and calm her fears, I said the stupidest thing that we doctors ever say, which is, "Just relax." Then, "Please just relax. This is, after all, just a routine procedure. This is how I make my living." Through clenched teeth came the reply, "Well it is certainly not how I make mine."

Stanley Marcus and the "Good Guys"

Every December for 25 years, Stanley Marcus hosted what he named the "Good Guys" Luncheon. No set criteria for inclusion were ever remotely clear to me. Mostly they were just people he liked, or who had qualities or achievements that he admired or wished to recognize. Sometimes Stanley used the occasion to make a statement, as when he placed the writer and aesthete Leon Harris at his right elbow – the place of honor – after Leon had made a very unflattering reference to Stanley in a just-published book. This was not to show forgiveness, in my view, but to show who the bigger man was. I don't recall Leon being there in subsequent years.

I was at the place of honor once, in 1976, the year after I had left private practice to become an Associate Dean at UT Southwestern Medical School. I had retained a small private practice with Stanley, of course, included. Stanley, with his usual discernment, felt that I would be too distracted by my new responsibilities to optimally function as his personal physician, so he had dismissed me with his customary grace, and had sought and accepted my recommendation for Paul "Brownie" Thomas to be his new physician. Placing me at his right – and including me in the list – was his way of bestowing favor and showing that I had not been personally rejected.

The list would change a bit each year, but there was a cadre of regulars, not all of whom I can recall for sure: Al Casey, nonpareil raconteur and boon companion, Stan's longtime insurance man, Sam Jaffe, Ted Strauss, brother of famous lawyer and democrat power broker, Bob Strauss, who also came in the early years, before he became Ambassador to Russia, an appointment that may have excited some envy in Stanley, an emotion he almost never evinced.

Bud Oglesby, a great architect, was also a regular, as was Bill Booziotis, another leading architect, friend and factotum to the affluent. The author/historian/journalist A.C. Green, developer Ken Hughes, Ray Nasher of North Park, and later Nasher Sculpture Garden and Museum fame, was as proud to be there as any of us. There was also Bob Wilson, first and permanently the best ever President of the local PBS outlet, and later a successful author and advertising executive. Also Jeffrey Weiss, quondam independent oil man with a flamboyant lifestyle, while it lasted, and a rare gift for personal friendships.

There were many others, perhaps 40 or more. Dr. Bryan Williams was an original and faithful attendee. Other regulars included longtime Chairman of Medicine, Dr. Donald Seldin, and later on, my former partner and close friend Dr. Jabez Galt. Jabez became the de facto secretary and archivist, doing annual minutes in style of Samuel Pepys. To the last meeting came Dr. Kern Wildenthal, the gifted, diffident and immensely successful longtime President of our Health Science Center. One favorite was the great, innovative automobile dealership mogul, Carl Sewell. Carl was, in a way, emblematic of qualities the "Good Guys" enjoyed.

Successful he was, but more important to the gathering, he brought a reliably really awful joke or two from the used car lot. Contrasted with his cherubic face and choirboy manner, the effect was hilarious – and unrepeatable. Bud Oglesby, who was so neat, quiet and, well, artistic, offered a milder but similar contrast. Remember that presidential campaign that was enlivened by the disastrous Gary Hart scandal? Bud reported that his saintly mother, nearing 90, had announced that Gary Hart was now the eighth dwarf, "Horny."

Roger Horchow, among Stanley's closest friends, told the story one year of how he put together his Tony-winning Broadway musical (based on "Girl Crazy"), "Crazy for You," and all that had been involved in getting the Gershwin heirs to sign off on the project. Roger's report ushered in the new, expurgated format brought about at the insistence of Stanley's wife, Linda. Times were changing, and Linda was wise. On her recommendation, anything sexist and chauvinistic was banned. Some of the jokes and comments, overheard by passersby in the hallway and by waiters and serving people, could well have gotten us all, particularly Stanley, in a heap of trouble.

Thereafter, the gatherings were still very interesting, but never quite as much fun as they had been in the first 15 or 20 years.

One new experimental program conforming to the new format featured the one female personality ever invited, political columnist Molly Ivins. Molly told two hilarious stories about her chum, Governor Ann Richards. One time Molly and the Governor were invited to a luncheon, probably at the Driskill Hotel in Austin, a weekly or monthly affair given by a bunch of good old boys in the Texas House of Representatives. After a half hour of listening to stories about big boobs and other off-color topics, there came a pause. Molly asked Ann if she had had any interesting experiences lately.

"Why yeah," Ann replied. "I was driving along Sixth Street just the other day and such a man I saw. I couldn't believe what I was seeing, the biggest balls I'd ever seen. They must have been as big as volleyballs."

In the other story, Ann, the incoming Treasurer of the state of Texas, was going through a reception line made up of state leaders shaking hands with several political powerbrokers. Ann was in line behind a newly elected black congressman, who we'll call Lester Smith. When his turn came to shake hands, one of the elitists, a notorious racist, asked the incoming congressman, "And what's your name, boy?"

Then came Ann's turn, "And what's your name and who might you be, little lady?" The answer came, "Why, I'm Mrs. Smith."

Despite Molly Ivins' stories, the experiment was not a success. For one thing, Stanley committed a rare social error: he seated Molly next to the other career journalist and author at the head table, A.C. Green. Two large egos, not unfriendly, exactly, just distant. The body language revealed all. The other problem was the fact that conservatives in the group were not charmed.

So that ended the co-ed experiment. Subsequent luncheons featured a topic or two and designated speakers. It was not like the jejune exuberance of the first years, but still very enjoyable.

For many years, the luncheon was held at the Dallas Club, an elegant downtown congress of businessmen and professionals. We began looking for the invitation in the fall. It usually arrived in October or November. We would convene at noon; Bloody Marys, screwdrivers, wine, and beer were served, and then came a meal, always good, but never the centerpiece of the event.

ALBERT D. ROBERTS, MD

Stanley would make a few remarks, introduce new members and offer some reflections on events of the past year. Then came the jokes and the narratives. One year we were bidden to offer limericks and originality was encouraged. I was a little surprised at so many in this group had no idea what a limerick was. Some fairly dreadful doggerel ensued.

One of the group's favorites was Neil Mallon, the wispy, puckish, octogenarian President Emeritus of Dresser Industries. Neil had two bits of doggerel that we all insisted he recite every year. One I remember well. Picture a frail, elderly man with a slightly quavering voice:

    The sexual drive of the camel
     is stronger than anyone thinks.
    In a fit of unbridled passion,
     one tried to make love to the sphinx.
    But the sphinx's nether posterior
    was filled with the sands of the Nile
    which accounts for the
    hump on the camel
    and the sphinx's inscrutable smile.

The second Mallon favorite, mostly forgotten, was about the Poetry Contest, wherein schoolboys were required to make a poem in rhyme ending with the word "Timbuktu." The first contestant offered a nice poem about a stately galleon, ending "destination, Timbuktu."

    A second contestant offered a different perspective:
    As Tim and I walked out to pass the time of day
    We spied three dusky maidens who seemed to smile our way.
    As they be three and we be two
    I bucked one and Tim bucked two.

Many of the members would not speak except to join in the lively table talk. One who did always speak was Cecil Greene, one of the legendary founders of Texas Instruments. Cecil was a regular well into his 90s, and he did ramble on a bit. Still, he's among those I recall best, particularly his insightful revelations about TI's early dealings in the Middle East – the Saudis, the Shah; and so on – and on and on…

A LIFETIME IN MEDICINE

One year, there was a recently retired admiral, a recent arrival in Dallas. Though he was only there the one time, departing soon for parts unknown, I remember him for his floridly handsome face and beautifully tailored suit, as well as for the joke he told:

It was during the Italian campaign, World War II. A German Oberst was killed and mistakenly sent to the Italian hell, where mortified and furious, he demanded to be transferred to the German hell to be with the rest of his men. So eventually, he was transferred, and the Italians were very glad to be rid of him. At the exchange point, his German compatriots asked him how he liked the Italian hell:

"Vell, it is not zo bad. Every day forced marches, full packs, river of shit, road full of ground glass. But you know the Italians: always running out of ground glass; never enough shit."

After an hour or so of this sort of thing, Stanley would close the proceedings, and we all would leave with our party favors – a handsome Neiman's tote bag containing six or eight items from the store. In later years, when Stanley was no longer President of Neiman's, a bag of Jabez Galt's prize-winning Mount Vernon, Texas, pecans was included. These small items, I suspect, were among the gifts that were not selling too well that season, but they were each beautifully, individually wrapped. Every Christmas at our house, the custom was for me to pass the grab bag around after all the presents had been opened. One year a piece retrieved by my mother-in-law, Mayme Truett, was a small notepad adorned with small pen and ink drawings of an orgy: several dozen small nude figures engaged in a graphic display of every imaginable sex act and position. The notepad heading was "Things to do Today." I snatched it away from Mayme before she saw what it was, and said, "Oh! Stanley meant this for me."

I kept the pad, and for years would use it to send personal notes to Stan. He always maintained that he had no idea how it got in there.

At the 25th "Good Guys" luncheon, Stanley ended it with a graceful little speech about how all things must come to an end. I am reasonably sure that he did not close it down due to foreseeing his own end – he was in good condition despite many medical issues and lived another several years. We all protested, and some vowed to perpetuate it, but deep down we knew he was right, and we never seriously tried to revive it.

Below is a contribution I made one year in honor of Stanley's 90th birthday:

> 90 CHEERS AND A FEW RHYMES FOR STANLEY
> First year in the majors for a young Ty Cobb
> Battleship Potemkin falls to a mob
> Invention of rayon
> First light by neon
> Picasso in Paris, his period pink.
> Freud in Vienna; just to think:
> His "Three Contributions to The Theory of Sex"
> Can barely excite, let alone vex
> A Vienna enchanted by Lehar and Strauss,
> And the tottering scandalous royal house.
> A Nobel for Koch, the one for lit.
> To an astonished Pole named Sienkiewick.
> Santayana publishes "Life of Reason"—
> 1905 is an astonishing season!
> So ruffles and flourishes; a blast from the horn!
> For 1905, the year Stanley is born!
> Now rejoice we Good Guys, gaudeamus!
> Let '95 be just as famous!
> Bill Booziotis, raise a toast
> Albert Casey, start the roast
> Is A.C. Greene? Is Marvin Wise?
> Is Dick a Hitt? Here's some advice:
> Hoist a beaker with Donald Seldin!
> Lorrie Marcus, sound the welkin
> Henry Miller, Rollin King
> Fisher, Mantz and Temerlin
> Raise your voices, make a fuss!
> Marcus Ginsburg, Henry Jacobus,
> Barton Tansky - pass the word:
> Let every member's heart be stirred!
> To Sewell and Walker, Baby Boomers—
> A glass to rectify your humors.
> E.G. Hamilton, Patrick Esquerre
> Cecil Green - let all be merry.

A LIFETIME IN MEDICINE

Pass the jug to Vincent Carrozza
And Irvin Jaffe. Heaven knows a
Sanguine heart and merry spirit
Shall praise the grape and never fear it.
Dunning, Galt, Hughes and Goldman,
Dayton, Williams, Woodward, Grossman
Set your tables on a roar,
And banish gloom forevermore.
Wake up, Bromberg—there's a chance
That Roger Horchow will do his dance!
Storey, Nasher, Jeffrey Weiss—
Carpe diem! in a trice
Before we know, the moment passes.
So Wilson, Pistor—fill your glasses,
Richard Marcus, Smith and Garrett—
A little quiet, if you can bear it—
While from Al Roberts who wrought these rhymes,
And from all good guys, the best of times
To Stanley Marcus, and all good cheer
Till we meet again, another year
To join together in ribald fun
And set our sights on ninety-one.

Stanley taught me many things in both medical practice and in life. He was critical and exacting. Although I never felt his lash, I knew from others that carelessness, incompetence, indifference or discourtesy could provoke a withering critique. But, as with another mentor, Dr. Seldin, the criticism was in service to the goal of excellence. The legendary eye for detail that he brought to all things great and small, he also focused from time to time on aspects of my medical practice, not the diagnosis and treatment part, but fairly often on how it was conducted. I saw what pleased him and what did not, and I benefited from so doing.

Some things we have never gotten right.

"Why do so many pills look alike?"

"Why can't you people consolidate your medical bills? If Bloomies can do it, why can't you?"

ALBERT D. ROBERTS, MD

The Doctor – Patient Dyad

In any medical practice involving substantial ongoing personal responsibility over time, physicians enter into a transforming dialogue with their patients and are themselves as much or more modified by the encounters as are the patients, who, for their part, little realize the effect that they're having on their doctors. When we are sad, depressed or just very tired, our patients lift our spirits, a benefit or dividend on the prior investments of empathy, time and effort, and a fund of favorable outcomes past. They also deflate us, bringing us back to earth if we become overconfident, careless or self-satisfied.

On a deeper level, the demands made by grappling with hard problems, difficult relationships and responsibilities sustained over time must deepen our personal understanding, broaden our self-knowledge and develop our character. To be sure, physicians must maintain personal integrity and professional standards at all times, and if they are wise, learn from their experiences. They must be ever attuned to the problem of closeness, by which I mean that spectrum between excessive familiarity on the one hand, and cold, alienating objectivity on the other. But I want to make the particular point here that when we accept the responsibilities for ongoing patient care, we are also consenting, knowingly or not, to be molded by the experience.

It has seemed to me that these innumerable daily interactions, compounded over decades, accrue an organicity of their own, become a third entity, "the practice."

For a career in medicine is not made nor a reputation founded on an occasional "star turn," the brilliant diagnosis or dramatic treatment success, though such things certainly help. No. It is like a coral reef. It is a structure built from the accumulation over time of thousands of small actions: patient listening, the unexpected follow-up phone call or bedside visit, a house call. Steadfastness in adversity. Good humor. Availability.

"Amo et fis," said Augustine of Hippo, which in the Augustinian context means, "Love God and do what you will." This has been historically misinterpreted as freedom to sin, as long as one believed. The good bishop Augustine requires us to love God so completely that we can do no wrong.

Perhaps in a secular age, a similar injunction might be applied to a profession: love law, or accounting, or economics, and do what you will. Or medicine.

A LIFETIME IN MEDICINE

Constant devotion to the profession of medicine cannot, finally, preserve us from error. But it does ennoble our efforts, enrich our lives and see us through to the end.

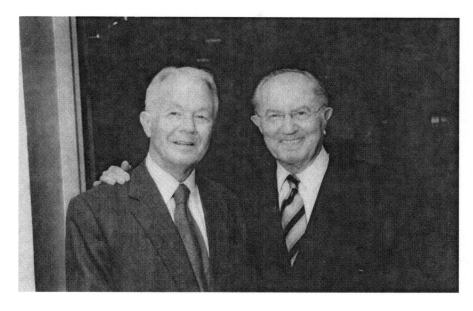

Dr. Don Seldin, right, pictured with me at my retirement celebration.

CPSIA information can be obtained at www.ICGtesting.com
Printed in the USA
BVOW02s0119120615

404323BV00001B/126/P